POTS SYNDROME

WHAT IT REALLY IS & WHY IT HAPPENS

Patrick Ussher

Copyright © Patrick Ussher (2017)

Disclaimer

Please note that the contents of this book are not intended as a substitute for medical advice or treatment. Any person with a medical condition requiring medical attention should consult a qualified medical practitioner. The author of this book does not accept any liability for injury, losses or damages which may occur as a result of following the recommendations made in this book.

Dedicated with all my love to Mum
(August 25th, 1950 - April 6th, 2015)
I kept my promise.

About the Author

Patrick Ussher followed the *Dynamic Neural Retraining System*, an intensive six-month limbic system rehabilitation program, to recover from POTS. After he recovered, he set about mapping the idea of POTS as a form of limbic system impairment onto pre-existing scientific research into the condition, to see if it could be the 'missing link' which could explain the root cause of the condition. This book is the result of that research.

Patrick was also part of the *Stoicism Today* project from its inception in 2012 until 2016, a collaboration of academics and psychotherapists which provided modernised Stoic resources based on the ancient Greco-Roman philosophy as a way of life. Patrick contributed to the development of three 'International Stoic Weeks' (2012-2014), which were widely featured in the media including on BBC Radio, and in newspapers such as *The Guardian*, *Forbes* and *The Telegraph*. Patrick edited the blog for the *Stoicism Today* project (https://blogs.exeter.ac.uk/stoicismtoday) from 2012 until 2016 and has also edited two books: *Stoicism Today: Selected Writings (Volumes One & Two)*. Patrick has a BA and MA in Classics from the University of Exeter, U.K., and currently lives in Dublin, Ireland.

Table of Contents

Introduction 1

Notes.. 8

Chapter One: Where We Are Now 9

Chapter Two: What is Really Going on in POTS
Syndrome & Why it Happens.. 33

Chapter Three: Explaining the Whole Elephant (or How
Limbic System Malfunction Can Explain Everything We
Know About POTS)... 61

Chapter Four: Rewiring the Limbic System & A
Biological Hypothesis for Recovery 89

Chapter Five: A Potential Protocol For Recovery and
Outline of a Trial to Test this Hypothesis.........................121

Addendum: General Points About Recovery and the
DNRS Program 143

Introduction

This book has two aims:

1. One aim is to present a new theory for the origins of POTS syndrome and, in light of this new theory, to suggest that it is possible to correct the underlying cause. The presentation of this hypothesis is primarily aimed at those medical researchers who work in the field of dysautonomia in the hope that they will see the merits in what is put forward, and design a research program to test the efficacy of the *Dynamic Neural Retraining System* (the 'DNRS') for POTS syndrome.

2. In addition, the book also aims to give hope to the person currently suffering from POTS syndrome that their condition may finally have an explanation and that, if they are convinced with that explanation (regardless of whether a research trial into the efficacy of limbic system rehabilitation for POTS has taken place), they may still be able to find an effective treatment in the form of the DNRS program. In line with this, this book also hopes to act as a guide for those using the DNRS program as a treatment specifically for POTS.

I wish to make clear at this point, however, that this book does not, in and of itself, present the step by step methods by which to treat the condition using neural retraining methods. This book is an hypothesis: it is not, in itself, a 'how to guide'. The limbic system rehabilitation program as offered by the DNRS is best placed to provide that guide. If you have POTS and you think that the thesis I am putting forward might point to the underlying cause of the condition, then the decision to pursue the DNRS as a treatment - whether through their DVD set or in-person program - will be a decision for you to make.

Let me say more so as to explain the rationale behind this book. I myself had POTS syndrome but I recovered using the *Dynamic Neural Retraining System*, an intensive six month 'brain rewiring' program. It was developed by Annie Hopper, who herself had a form of brain impairment known as 'Multiple Chemical Sensitivity' (or 'MCS'), but recovered from that condition by applying specific brain rewiring exercises which later became the basis for the DNRS program. Hopper developed that program for those suffering with MCS but later found that it could also work for those with POTS. I was one of those with POTS for whom it worked (although, interestingly, I had also become moderately sensitive to chemicals before taking the program).

Once I had recovered, I set about attempting to understand why a 'brain rewiring' program might have led to my recovery, and that of others, from POTS. I read widely about POTS syndrome and it seemed to me that the principal findings on the condition to date could be explained once the idea of a physical brain impairment in the limbic system was taken into account. I became more and more certain that I had not recovered as the result of a 'placebo effect' but rather that brain dysfunction was indeed the 'missing link', the factor which rendered the 'mysterious' nature of POTS explicable.

I do not have any medical qualifications nor do I have a background in science. I am aware that as a result I present the hypothesis in quite a broad and general way. There are certain claims I make which are based on 'lived experience' (both of myself and of others whose progress I have followed in their own recovery journeys). There are other times when I make points which are (I hope) 'scientific common sense'. However, I admit that I may have got some things wrong even if the hypothesis is, as I believe it is, along the right lines. I hope the reader will forgive any errors made and remember that my real hope is that a researcher may take this hypothesis on one day, refine it and make it as 'scientifically sound' as it needs to be. Although I do try to write throughout with a degree of certainty, I am not at all tied to individual points I make if scientific investigation shows them to be wrong or misplaced in some way.

Let me say a few more words of introduction. The fact that there are so many physiological problems occurring in the POTS patient - from tachycardia to NET protein deficiency to low aldosterone to mast cell activation problems - has often made it appear a 'mysterious' condition to both researcher and patient alike. It is, simply put, very hard to identify what must be the root cause when there are so many varied and often seemingly disparate symptoms. Prof. Raj, of the University of Calgary, himself a specialist in the field of dysautonomia, makes a very good point in this regard. He has described the attempt to understand POTS as being akin to the task of several blind men attempting to identify an elephant in front of them.[1] Depending on where they touch, they come up with different answers. Is it a wall? A snake? A rope? A spear, tree or fan? The same is true of POTS, depending on which aspects of the POTS patient one studies. Is it a form of extreme deconditioning? A form of neuropathy? A form of blood vessel dysfunction? A cardiac problem? All of these, and many more, have been suggested, by both medical researchers and patient groups.

I believe that the elephant analogy holds true. Perhaps we have been like the blind men, unable to see what is actually in front of us. Indeed, rather than focussing on different parts of the 'elephant' separately, we need some way of taking the whole 'elephant' into account and of explaining why it is acting the way it is *as a whole*. And that is the aim of this book: to present an hypothesis which explains the 'whole elephant'. I believe that so far research, although it has identified various crucial physiological problems, has been looking at the branches of the tree rather than at its

---

[1] See mins. 22.00 ff. of Prof. Raj's talk 'Connecting the dots between EDS and POTS', accessible at:
www.YouTube.com/watch?v=srUJRRihvsE

roots. I argue in this book that there is *one* root cause and that its treatment can and should lead to the return to health of all the POTS 'branches'.

I believe that limbic system impairment - a very physical impairment to that part of the brain - can explain the key findings in POTS to date, including NET protein deficiency (the root cause of blood vessel constriction problems upon standing up in POTS patients and resulting elevated heart rate), low aldosterone and sodium retention levels (the main contributory factors to low blood volume in POTS patients), mast cell activation problems and much more besides, including conditions that often overlap with POTS, such as Fibromyalgia, Irritable Bowel Syndrome (and other digestive issues), Chronic Fatigue Syndrome and Multiple Chemical Sensitivity. The case of Multiple Chemical Sensitivity is especially important. For, even though MCS has been rarely mentioned in connection with POTS up until now, the DNRS was actually originally developed, as I mentioned above, as a treatment for that condition. What was found subsequently however is that some patients with both MCS and POTS who followed the DNRS program actually recovered from *both* conditions, a fact which suggests a shared neurological origin in the limbic system. Sometimes important advances in scientific understanding happen 'by accident' and I believe this to be one of those cases.

And the link between MCS and POTS is significant for other reasons too. This is because MCS is *obviously* a neurological condition affecting the limbic system.

Why? MCS usually (but not always) occurs after some kind of chemical poisoning and leads the parts of the brain which process smell - which are firmly rooted in the limbic system - to rewire themselves into a chronic state of hypervigilance following that trauma, leading the sufferer's sense of smell to change drastically. Indeed, the person with MCS soon finds all chemicals to be noxious (in some cases to the point of anaphylactic shock). The reason this is obviously neurological is that it is clearly a condition that affects sensory perception and sensory perception is, of course, processed neurologically by the limbic system. Given this, the fact that the DNRS has led to the recovery of those with both MCS *and* POTS points to the fact that both share a similar neurological origin, even if the reasons why either condition might develop are different and even if different parts of the limbic system are adversely affected primarily. I will have more to say on the link between MCS and POTS in the main argument of the book.

The book also takes seriously the significance of there usually being a traumatic triggering event (understood broadly to include physical traumas, such as a viral illness or Lyme disease) that precedes POTS syndrome. Indeed, there is a medical consensus that POTS is preceded by a traumatic event or that it can build progressively as a result of more insidious traumas over a longer period. However, the significance of the condition being preceded by a traumatic event has not, I believe, been grappled with yet fully. Given the fact that there usually is a preceding trauma and that this is an observable constant, it really must hold the key to understanding the true nature of the condition. I believe that it does and that these traumas can explain in very clear ways, as we shall see, why POTS is actually a form of limbic system impairment.

On this book's companion website (www.whatpotsreallyis.net), the reader will find additional evidence which supports the book's main ideas, in the form of testimonials by those who have used the DNRS as an effective treatment for POTS. I hope that this 'anecdotal evidence' will in turn inspire others to consider using the DNRS as a treatment for their own POTS and also that it may inspire researchers to investigate the DNRS as a possibly effective treatment for the condition.

Two other expressions of gratitude. I would like to express my admiration for Annie Hopper for her work in designing the DNRS program so skilfully with limbic system impairment in mind. Without the courage to have developed it first of all to treat MCS, it might never have come to pass that its efficacy for POTS would have become known. And I would also like to express my admiration for Lauren Dinkel, one of the first with POTS and MCS to recover using the DNRS, and whose inspiring website (http://wheelchairorollerblades.com) I stumbled across when I was unwell and seeking treatment options. Before I started the DNRS program, I wrote to her: 'Lauren, let's beat POTS!'

Here's to hoping that we may have done just that.

Notes

A. Contact information for the DNRS can be found here: https://retrainingthebrain.com/contact-us/

B. The Book's Youtube Channel ('What POTS Really Is')

The principal parts of the book are also contained in a one hour YouTube talk, and a variety of other shorter talks on the channel also consider other aspects of the ideas put forward in the book.

C. Gathering Evidence for the Efficacy of the DNRS for POTS

If you have used the DNRS for at least six months to treat POTS, please consider blogging about your experience or creating a Youtube video.

Please also consider submitting a written testimonial of your experience of using the DNRS as a treatment for POTS to the book's companion website (www.what potsreallyis.net)
via the email whatpotsreallyis@icloud.com. I hope to publish a second edition of this book in the future which will contain testimonials of those who have treated their POTS effectively by following the DNRS - your testimonial could be one of them.

I welcome emails from readers of the book. Please note, however, that I may not be able to answer every email due to other work and time constraints.

Chapter One: Where We Are Now

The new hypothesis in this book takes the most significant existing scientific findings concerning POTS syndrome and attempts to explain them by reference to a hitherto unconsidered root cause. In order, therefore, to put forward this new hypothesis, we must first consider the research on the condition to date. In this chapter, I outline the main aspects of the current medical research on POTS syndrome, including a discussion of the acronym itself, the status of the condition as a 'syndrome', current thinking on what kinds of events tend to 'trigger' the condition and typical methods used to treat it. I will then proceed to the most important part of this chapter which will entail considering, in detail, the two main hypotheses to date as to its biological causes, namely that of 'deconditioning' and that of 'NET protein deficiency', thereby laying the groundwork for the rest of this book.[2] I note here that I am aware that there are other

---

[2] In writing the sections of this book concerning pre-existing research on POTS, I have found the following two resources especially helpful. First of all, Prof. Raj's 2013 overview of POTS published in the journal, *Circulation* (accessible here: http://circ.ahajournals.org/content/127/23/2336.long) and, second, the thorough collection of articles in the third edition of *The Primer on the Autonomic Nervous System,* edited by Robertson, Biaggioni, Burnstock, Low and Paton. I also note here that, throughout this book, I do not always reference page numbers, but the paper or chapter number,of the article or paper in question.

hypotheses that have been put forward regarding the condition's cause. There are, however, good reasons for limiting our discussion to NET deficiency and to deconditioning at this point. This is because both of these theories potentially relate most obviously of all to the pronounced heart rate increase upon standing that one sees in the POTS patient. In terms, therefore, of explaining why this cardiac elevation is present, it makes sense to focus on these two theories first of all. However, other aspects of research into what is going wrong at a physiological level in POTS patients will also be considered in chapter three.

POTS Syndrome: An Overview of its Symptoms and the Significance of the Term 'Syndrome'

Let us start our discussion where most discussions of POTS syndrome start: by explaining what the acronym stands for. The letters "POTS" do not, in fact, seek to do anything other than describe some of the more pronounced symptoms of the condition. Let's consider each word in turn:

- 'Postural': This implies that the symptoms are particularly manifest depending on the body's position or 'posture'.

- 'Orthostatic': This defines in what kind of posture these symptoms are most manifest, namely when the body is 'orthostatic' or 'upright'

This only pertains to electronic resources I made use of when the print page number was not available. For other works, for example, Annie Hopper's *Wired for Healing*, I include page numbers.

- 'Tachycardia': This refers to the fact that, upon standing, the patient has a fast heartbeat.

Taken together, we may say simply that *when the patient stands up their heart beats unusually faster than normal*. We can add that the standard medical definition suggests that the heart rate of the POTS patient increases by 30 beats or more from supine to standing within the space of 10 minutes. Prof. Raj describes these essential criteria as follows:

"The most striking physical feature of POTS is the severe tachycardia that develops on standing from a supine position. Blood pressure and heart rate must be measured in both postures and should be taken not only immediately after standing but also at 2, 5 and 10 minutes as occasionally patients have a delayed tachycardia. Normal subjects commonly develop a transient tachycardia within the 1st minute of standing that should not be mistaken for POTS. A sustained heart rate increase ≥30 beats per minute is considered diagnostic of orthostatic tachycardia."[3]

For example, if a patient has a resting heart rate of 85 BPM (beats per minute) when lying down and this increases to, say, 115 BPM (or more) upon standing, then that person meets the diagnostic criteria for POTS. There is, as many readers will know from personal experience, a particular kind of test that measures this 'heart rate differential between supine and standing' with particular accuracy, and that is the 'tilt-table test'.

---

[3] Raj, 2013.

It is, of course, *normal* for the heart rate to increase upon standing up in everyone, *for the heart has to work harder to pump blood to the brain in response to the extra work of being upright.* However, in the person *without* POTS syndrome, the heart rate usually only increases between 10 to 20 beats from supine to standing, not 30, 40, or even 50 beats more, as is seen in the case of the POTS patient. As Prof. Raj has written of the heart rate increase upon standing in the healthy person: the '...assumption of upright posture results in a 10-20 beat per minute increase in heart rate.'[4] Similarly, Wieling and Groothuis write that under normal circumstances:

"Orthostatic pooling of blood begins almost immediately upon the change from the supine to the upright posture and is estimated to total 300-800 mL; the bulk of total change occurs within the first 5-10 seconds. In humans, orthostatic adjustments are provided by an effective set of blood pressure regulatory mechanisms. They maintain blood pressure at an appropriate level for perfusion of the vital organs, even for the brain, which is located above the heart. To achieve this, the regulatory systems increase heart rate, cardiac contractility and vascular tone to stabilize blood pressure at the level of the heart and brain."[5]

The key difference in the case of the POTS patient, therefore, is that something causes an 'extra' increase

---

[4] Raj, 2013.

[5] From *The Primer on the Autonomic Nervous System* (eds. Robertson, Biaggioni, Burnstock, Low and Paton), 2011, chapter 39. [Henceforth: *ANS Primer*, 2011].

in heart rate above and beyond that which should occur anyway. Later in this chapter, we shall consider the two principal theories put forward for why this is the case.

However, it is important to note, as any patient with POTS will know, that the condition involves more than just a quick heart beat. Rather, there is a range of symptoms which can make daily life debilitating and, in some cases, nigh-on-impossible. As Low and Sandroni write:

"The following orthostatic symptoms occurred in >75% of subjects: light-headedness/dizziness, lower extremity or diffuse weakness, disequilibrium, tachycardia, shakiness…other autonomic symptoms were dry eyes or mouth, gastrointestinal complaints of bloating, early satiety, nausea, pain and alternation of diarrhoea and constipation. Fatigue is a significant complaint in about half of patients."[6]

The wide range of symptoms that the POTS patient feels should be an indication that the condition is more than just a heart problem, as it is sometimes mistakenly viewed. Rather, this is a condition which affects many functions of the body. It is also arguably regrettable that, for a condition in which patients feel unwell nearly all of the time that their condition should be termed 'POTS', something which implies that the problems only occur upon the action of standing up. This could not be further from the truth and this is only one reason why, as we shall see, the term 'POTS' is

---

[6] *ANS Primer* (2011), Chapter 106.

inadequate in describing the condition's root cause: rather, the term is merely a descriptor of certain quantifiable aspects of the condition.

This brings us to the significance of terming POTS a 'syndrome'. For, calling a condition a 'syndrome' implies that the root cause of that condition is currently unknown, even if its symptoms can be quantified and analysed. This further implies that once the root cause has been identified, the condition can be renamed more accurately. At the moment, however, the importance of the word 'syndrome' has often been lost. Amongst many of the heart-wrenching videos of POTS patients online, you often find the idea put forward that they have a 'heart condition that affects my ability to stand up'. When this happens, the significance of the word 'syndrome' is lost, and the word is *really* significant. It would be more accurate to say: 'I have a condition, the cause and cure for which is currently unknown, but some of its most pronounced symptoms include a high heart rate upon standing.' It is important that the acronym 'POTS' is not used as a definition of the illness itself but rather as a diagnostic tool for a collection of a certain set of symptoms the cause of which is as yet unknown.

Current Modes of Treatment

This book is not intended to be an overview of current treatment protocols nor would it be appropriate for me to focus on them as I do not have any medical training. I mention these treatments only briefly here, primarily as doing so sets the scene for further discussion later of other aspects of the condition.

Current treatments focus on alleviating the patient's symptoms, primarily through attempts to increase the patient's blood volume, so as to stabilise blood pressure, but also on lowering the patient's heart rate through the use of beta-blockers (typically propranolol in small doses). Other commonly used drugs are midodrine, which in other contexts is normally given to elderly patients to increase blood pressure, and also Flurinef, which is a synthetic replacement of the hormone aldosterone, about which we will have more to say later and which, for various reasons, effectively raises blood volume. Patients are also advised to add plenty of salt to their food and drink extra water so as to increase blood volume further. In addition, many patients begin a cardiovascular reconditioning program with, once more, the aim of increasing blood volume (as a result of improved cardiac performance). The rationale behind all of these measures, given what we currently know, is clearly well-founded - low blood volume is a significant problem for POTS patients. These approaches often do lead to a return of (relative) functionality in a considerable number of patients, but rarely to the remission of the illness.

What 'Triggers' POTS?

In turning now to the reasons POTS comes about, the key point is that there is usually a 'triggering event'. You do not 'catch' POTS in the same way you might catch an infectious disease. Rather, it seems to be triggered by something which *happens* to you, and you can develop the condition whether you were previously healthy or not. There is widespread agreement among researchers that the following events nearly always precede POTS and as such seem to 'trigger' it:

- a virus, such as mononucleosis or another illness, such as Lyme disease[7]
- a surgery, serious physical injury or pregnancy
- a traumatic event, whether emotional, physical or psychological

The link between all of these seemingly disparate kinds of traumatic events and the onset of POTS is, on the face of it, rather puzzling. How can so many different things lead potentially to the *same* condition? However, as we shall see in chapter two, there is a link and it is central to the nature of the condition. Indeed, the idea of POTS being preceded by a triggering traumatic event is central to the whole hypothesis I will be putting forward.

Underlying Biological Mechanisms of POTS: Two Schools of Thought

We now turn to the biological mechanisms seen in POTS and, in particular, to considering two of the main hypotheses that have been put forward as to the condition's biological cause, i.e. investigations into

---

[7] Indeed, Low and Sandroni (*ANS Primer*, chapter 106) note that around 50% of patients have an antecedent viral illness.

what has actually gone wrong at a physiological level in the patient's body. Consideration of these mechanisms is essential to the new hypothesis I am putting forward as one of them can, I believe, be explained by that hypothesis. The two theories I wish to discuss are the following:

1. 'The 'Deconditioning' theory
2. The 'NET [Norepinephrine Reuptake Transporter] protein deficiency' theory

Both theories, as we shall see, have considerable evidence in support of their claims. But only one of them can be right, in terms of the root cause of the condition (or in terms of *pointing towards* the root cause), for the two theories could not be further apart from each other.

As I mentioned at the start of this chapter, I am aware there are a number of other theories often put forward regarding the biological origins of POTS syndrome. I focus on only these two here as both deconditioning and NET protein deficiency relate most obviously, as we shall see, to the elevated heart rate seen in POTS upon standing. Other theories regarding the biological origins of POTS syndrome will be considered in chapter three. There is, however, another benefit to focussing just on these two theories as to do so cuts through much of the haze that obfuscates the condition - there are dozens of 'causes' you can find mentioned online but this haze can be lifted by focussing on those possible causes which we *definitely* know affect POTS patients. Indeed, we know from research that NET protein deficiency affects *all* POTS patients and we know that cardiac deconditioning also affects *all* POTS patients. (as we shall see from studies we shall consider shortly). On the other hand, sometimes you find, for example, "chiari malformation" (structural defects in the lower parts of the skull) mentioned as causing POTS but this most likely only affects a very small number of patients. Therefore, in sticking with cardiovascular deconditioning and NET protein deficiency, I am focussing on the most applicable evidence. Indeed, if the root cause of POTS is to be identified then it must be something which *all* POTS patients share, not just a few of them.

Let us now consider each of these theories in more detail.

The 'Deconditioning' Theory

In essence, the deconditioning theory posits that the POTS patient has a very low level of cardiovascular fitness. The basic thought behind the physical deconditioning theory goes something like this. For some reason beyond their control, the patient has a period of prolonged bed rest. After this period of enforced inactivity, the body's cardiovascular system becomes compromised. Levine, who is the principal researcher into deconditioning in POTS patients, argues that there is '...the presence of cardiac atrophy......along with reduced blood volume...as key components of the pathogenesis of this syndrome'.[8] In

---

[8] Levine (2012), 3496.

other words, the argument goes that the heart has become smaller, weaker and, as a result, less effective at maintaining a strong blood volume, and that these factors are the primary reasons behind POTS. Levine notes that a smaller heart and reduced blood volume are physiological changes that are also usually 'observed after long-term bed rest',[9] as might be seen, for example, following illness, injury or pregnancy. In sum, some kind of event leads 'to a period of prolonged bed rest...often leading to profound deconditioning' and '...deconditioning has a profound effect on heart morphology and function as well as blood and plasma volume.'[10] Indeed, Levine makes the case for renaming POTS syndrome 'Grinch Syndrome' after the folk-tale character who (from a metaphorical and emotional point of view) had a small heart.[11] Levine has developed an intensive cardiovascular rehabilitation programme for those with POTS syndrome. As utilised in one of Levine's trials, it is described as follows:

"Patients started a "personalized" exercise training program for 3 months after baseline testing... Three heart rate zones (e.g., recovery, base pace, and maximal steady-state) were identified based upon the maximal steady-state heart rate and resting heart rate. During the initial month of endurance training, patients engaged in base pace training with a calculated target heart rate of 75% intensity of their personal maximum intensity level. Sessions were prescribed 2-4 times per

---

[9] *Ibid.*

[10] Levine (2011), 76.

[11] Levine (2010), 2864.

week initially for 30-45 min per session using a recumbent bike, rowing, or swimming. The exercise protocol for this study was specifically tailored to POTS patients by requiring exercise to be performed in a semi-recumbent position for the initial 4-6 weeks of training. The protocol gradually introduced a more upright posture over the course of the 3-month time frame, allowing upright walking activity in the beginning of the third training month."[12]

The results after following this three month protocol were encouraging: both blood volume and heart size increased,[13] and, more importantly, from the data one can see that the average heart rate 'supine to standing differential' decreased considerably in patients (by around 9 beats on average).[14] For example, let's say one participant's heart rate increased by around 34 beats from supine to standing before the exercise protocol. After the protocol, that person's heart rate might only have increased by around 25 beats, taking them outside the diagnostic criterion for POTS of + 30 beats. For one of the trials Levine conducted this improvement in cardiovascular fitness meant that '...ten out of 17 participants no longer met criteria for

---

[12] Levine (2011), 74-75.

[13] See Levine (2010), 2866: "Left ventricular mass and end-diastolic volume increased by 12% and 8% after training, resulting in significant cardiac remodeling. The heart became much larger and probably more distensible after exercise training. Blood and plasma volumes also increased markedly after training. Ten (53%) of 19 patients no longer met criteria for POTS after completion of the 3-month exercise training program and thus were cured."

[14] See the graphs in Levine, 2010, 2011, 2012.

POTS post-training,'[15] leading to the suggestion that these patients were now 'cured' of POTS, but it was also noted that the underlying cardiovascular '...pathophysiology improved, but did not completely normalize' and that '...what levels of physical activity must be maintained in patients with POTS to achieve and maintain normal functional capacity is uncertain; however we speculate that a lifetime adherence to an active life-style will be necessary'.[16] In other words, even if the deconditioning theory is correct, three months might not be enough for a complete cure: you may have to keep up the intensive exercise for the rest of your life.

In sum, the deconditioning theory suggests that the patient is profoundly unfit following a period of bed rest and needs to be mindful of recovering fitness and maintaining it for the rest of his life.

Let us now turn to the next theory, that of 'NET protein deficiency'. As will be immediately grasped, this theory is the 'polar opposite' from the 'deconditioning theory' to the point that only *one* of them can really point to the biological cause. They are both talking about very different things.

NET protein deficiency

One uniting feature to have been discovered in nearly every POTS patient is the fact that their blood stream contains more of the hormone 'adrenalin' than is

---

[15] Levine (2010), 75.
[16] Levine 2012, 3503.

normal. Adrenalin is the 'fight or flight' hormone and it is also known as 'norepinephrine'. I add that the POTS patient has more norepinephrine in the blood stream than the person without POTS whether in supine *or* standing positions, although there is more in the latter. As Raj points out: 'The supine norepinephrine is often high normal in patients with POTS, while the upright norepinephrine is usually elevated (>600 pg/ml), a reflection of the exaggerated neural sympathetic tone that is present in these patients while upright.'[17] Indeed, some POTS patients will, as Raj elaborates, have 'extremely high' levels of adrenalin in their blood stream, over 1000 pg/mL in some cases, whereas the normal upper limit in those without POTS is just 475 pg/mL. It is for these reasons that POTS has been termed a 'hyperadrenergic' condition, i.e. the level of adrenalin in the blood stream is deemed to be far too much, or 'hyper'.

Why should it be that the POTS patient has more adrenalin floating around in their blood than the healthy person? Why is it that they can become, in other words, 'hyper-adrenergic'? And why does this happen especially when the patient is upright? The answer is crucial and is to be found in considering the role of a special protein, called the NET protein, and how it does not function properly in the person with POTS.

---

[17] Raj, 2013.

The NET protein functioning well

Before we can see how NET protein deficiency leads to a hyperadrenergic state, we need first to understand how the NET protein functions in the healthy person without POTS. I add that this section is rather complex and may only make sense once it has all been read through. Please read it slowly: it is crucial to the main ideas I am putting forward.

The NET protein stands for the '**N**or**e**pinephrine Reuptake **T**ransporter Protein'. Remember at this point that norepinephrine and adrenalin are the *same* substance and that, in that sense, the NET protein could easily also be called the 'Adrenalin Reuptake Transporter Protein'. From this name, we can tell that the function of the protein has something to do with 'reuptaking' adrenalin. But what does this actually mean? And why would this protein need to 'reuptake' adrenalin anyway?

We all know the feeling of adrenalin being released in response to stressful situations but what many of us are unaware of is the fact that adrenalin is a crucial hormone for overall health which is in fact being used by the body all of the time. For our purposes, it is important to note that the body makes use of adrenalin *whenever we stand up*. In particular, it makes use of the inherent ability of adrenalin to constrict (or tighten) blood vessels (this process of blood vessel constriction is called 'vasoconstriction'). This is in contrast to the 'opening' of blood vessels that occurs when the body is in a relaxed, supine position (this process is called 'vasodilation'). Why does the body constrict the blood vessels upon standing? The answer is that it does so because it leads to a more efficient process in which the overall area that the heart's pumping must fill is reduced. In other words, the 'tightening' of the blood vessels upon standing leads to a lower overall 'area' of blood in the body which the heart can more easily cope with in pumping blood throughout that overall area. As just mentioned, adrenalin is the substance that is capable of this blood vessel tightening, but it can't do this on its own. Rather, it needs help.

This is where the NET protein comes in. Unpicking the acronym will help show us why. 'Norepinephrine' refers to adrenalin, 'reuptake' refers to its ability to 'recycle' this adrenalin and 'transporter', to transport the hormone to and from storage in nearby cells.[18] In other words, the NET protein aims to 'capture' adrenaline that is nearby in the blood stream, store it in nearby cells, and then 'draw down' that stored adrenalin when the body requires it. And, as we have just seen, the body requires adrenalin for the process of vasoconstriction whenever we stand up. This is where the function of NET comes in: it aims to recycle adrenalin easily and efficiently so that blood vessel constriction can happen whenever required.

To put all of the above into simpler English: *there are countless NET proteins in your body whose job it is to recycle adrenalin so that your blood vessels can constrict*

---

[18] Goldstein, *ANS Primer*, Chapter 6: 'NE (norepinehprine) is inactivated mainly by uptake into cells, with subsequent intracellular metabolism or storage. Reuptake into nerve terminals...via the cell membrane NET is the predominant means of terminating the actions of released NE'.18

easily and efficiently upon standing. Ideally, when you stand up, this process is smooth, easy and efficient.

In the POTS patient, however, it is a different story.

When NET Ceases to Do Its Job: the Role of NET Deficiency in POTS

We know something has gone wrong with the NET protein in POTS patients as a result of groundbreaking advancements thanks, especially, to an Australian study, led by E. Lambert. Lambert et al., proved in 2008 that in POTS patients the NET protein has ceased to work properly. As Lambert puts it: 'Western blot analysis of NET protein extracted from forearm vein biopsies in patients with POTS...demonstrated a decrease in the expression of NET protein...'[19] The NET protein, in the POTS patient, therefore has become 'deficient'. How deficient? The basic difference between NET function in the normal person and in the POTS patient is as follows: *in the healthy person NET recycles 80%-90% of available adrenalin whereas in the POTS patient only between 40-60% of the available adrenalin is recycled.*[20]

What is the effect of this NET deficiency on the patient? In short, it is responsible, as a knock-on effect, for the

---

[19] See bibliography at the end of this chapter.

[20] For more details of healthy NET function and NET deficiency in POTS, see mins. 49.00-55.00 of this excellent Youtube lecture by Prof. Carrie Burdzinski: 'Postural Orthostatic Tachycardia Syndrome (POTS), Dysautonomia and the Autonomic Nervous System' (www.youtube.com/watch?v=faScrmgKcWg).

elevated heart rate upon standing. In essence, the effect of this NET deficiency on the patient is twofold:

i) the adrenalin that is not stored in nearby cells by NET instead remains in the bloodstream causing extra shakiness, light-headedness, a feeling of being 'on edge' and, of course, increased heart rate (as contact between adrenalin and the heart causes the latter to beat faster). This is the direct link between NET deficiency and the hyperadrenergic state of the POTS patient, i.e. the main reason why there is so much adrenalin in the blood stream of POTS patients.

ii) as the NET protein is deficient it is also unable to do its job of constricting the blood vessels properly upon standing. Rather it is only somewhat successful in this task and the blood vessels no longer constrict fully upon standing up. Instead, *they remain partially open*. The result of this is that the heart has to beat even faster in order to circulate the blood around the whole body: the wider the blood vessels upon standing, the greater the total 'space' in which blood must be pumped around the body, and the faster the heart must beat.

All of this essentially explains why the heart beats faster in the POTS patient upon standing up: the extra adrenalin is, from the point of view of the heart, an 'external factor' that forces it to beat faster against its wishes, whilst the widening of the blood vessels is, again from the point of view of the heart, an 'internal factor' by which the heart 'senses', whenever you stand up, the need to pump faster to keep the blood in full circulation around an expanded overall area. From this, it is clear that, despite what is sometimes thought, POTS syndrome is not primarily a cardiac condition. There is nothing intrinsically wrong with your heart that causes the problem (although in some cases, the extra strain on the heart might cause its own problems). Rather the heart is trying to do its best both to keep you conscious and to keep the blood flowing to where it should be. It is hampered, however, by the external factor of the extra presence of adrenalin and the internal factor of widened blood vessels, both of which stem from the NET proteins being unable to do their job.

These two problem areas also explain several other symptoms felt in the POTS patient. The 'adrenalin seepage' explains why POTS patients feel considerable 'somatic' anxiety. By this I mean 'sensations of anxiety in the body' as opposed to 'psychological anxiety'. Prof. Raj puts it this way: '...much of the (psychological) anxiety attributed to patients with POTS might be due to a misinterpretation of their physical symptoms.'[21] However, I add that the POTS patient may also have 'associated anxiety', i.e. understandable anxiety about having such a condition, in addition to feeling anxious because of the extra adrenalin floating around as a result of NET protein deficiency.

---

[21] Raj, 2013.

The second feature which NET protein deficiency explains is why there is more adrenalin in the blood stream of the POTS patient *upon standing* than whilst in the supine position. This is because the NET protein is only really called upon to do its work when someone stands up. When you are supine, your blood vessels do not need to be constricted and, concurrently, the NET protein does not need to do its work. But once the POTS patient stands up, the fact that the NET protein cannot recycle the available adrenalin properly, leading it to spill over into the blood stream, explains why the problems are particularly manifest upon standing. In other words, the POTS patient feels shakier upon standing as the deficient protein in question's primary work only occurs when someone stands up.

The third feature which this two-fold dysfunction explains in a sizeable minority of POTS patients is fainting. For, in extreme cases, the NET protein becomes so deficient that it hardly works at all. The blood vessels in these cases become *so* wide that, upon standing, the heart simply cannot beat fast enough to maintain blood flow to the brain and as a result the patient faints.

Why does the NET protein become deficient?

There was, understandably, a high level of excitement amongst medical researchers upon discovering the role of NET deficiency in POTS: at last we have found the main reason why things have gone so wrong! The question which then emerged was: *why does the NET protein no longer work properly*? Following initial findings at Vanderbilt University, work began there in earnest to find a genetic reason for NET deficiency: perhaps POTS patients were 'fated' in their DNA code to have deficient NET proteins. The genetics of hundreds of patients with POTS were studied. Was it found that an aberrant gene could be blamed for POTS?

In a word: no. With the exception of one family who carried an aberrant gene the other hundreds of patients considered gave no indication of any genetic change whatsoever. As the Vanderbilt website notes: 'For several years, we looked for this (genetic) mutation in other POTS patients. We have not found any other non-related patients to have this same loss of function mutation.' [22] Whatever the cause of NET deficiency is, therefore, it is not something 'fated' to happen to an unlucky few. No other reason for the breakdown in NET deficiency has, as yet, been put forward. We can conclude this section therefore with the simple claim that there must be *some* reason for NET deficiency, and that that reason is not genetic but environmental. It cannot be the case that the NET protein would just break down 'of its own accord', but rather that it breaks down *for some other reason entirely*. We will consider what this reason might be in the next chapter.

---

[22] See:
www.mc.vanderbilt.edu/root/vumc.php?site=adc&doc=43572

Conclusion: Two Very Different Theories

The 'deconditioning' argument and the 'NET protein deficiency' argument are clearly two very *different* theories. Indeed, they could not be further apart from each other. For this reason, common sense dictates that, despite the fact that there is strong evidence to support both theories, *only one of them can be correct* as to the biological cause as rather different mechanisms are indicated in both. For reasons I shall expand upon in the next chapter, I believe the NET protein deficiency argument to be the theory which is along the right lines, whereas the deconditioning theory describes an important clinical feature of POTS patients but is not the cause of the condition.

Key Points of Chapter One

In this chapter, we have considered the salient features of POTS syndrome, along with why the term 'POTS' is, at best, only a temporary descriptor. The term currently only describes some of the condition's symptoms, but it does not point to its cause, although this fact can sometimes be forgotten. We have also considered the fact that there is a 'triggering event' prior to the illness, whether a traumatic psychological or physical event or some kind of illness. With the exception of the deconditioning theory, no other theory has as yet been put forward as to why a triggering event might, in particular, be a catalyst for POTS syndrome.

Finally, we have discussed the two principal theories for POTS syndrome, namely that it is a result of profound cardiovascular weakening following a period of bed rest and that it is the result of a faulty NET protein, which causes the blood vessels to stay partially open upon standing and for adrenalin to 'seep out' into the blood stream. We have also considered how only one of these theories can point to *the* biological cause, given the fact that they are so different from each other.

Further Reading & Viewing:

1. For an excellent overview of the condition and of pre-existing research on it, see:

    - Raj., S. *The Postural Orthostatic Tachycardia Syndrome. Pathophysiology, Diagnosis & Management 2013* - http://circ.ahajournals.org/content/127/23/2336.full (referenced in this book as "Raj (2013)")

    In addition, Prof. Raj presents another excellent overview of the condition in the following YouTube lecture: *Connecting the Dots Between EDS and POTS*, - www.YouTube.com/watch?v=srUJRRihvsE .

    The following talk by Prof. Carrie Burdzinski, *Postural Orthostatic Tachycardia Syndrome (POTS), Dysautonomia, and the Autonomic Nervous System,* is superb in its detail and organisation - www.youtube.com/watch?v=faScrmgKcWg

For a comprehensive collection of articles on the autonomic nervous system, including several on POTS, see: *Primer on the Autonomic Nervous System*, Eds. Robertson, Biaggioni, Burnstock, Low and Paton, Academic Press, 2011 (referenced in this book as *ANS Primer*, chapter no. XX)

2. For a summary of the Australian NET deficiency paper, see:

> - Lambert, E., et al., *Altered sympathetic nervous reactivity and norepinephrine transporter expression in patients with postural tachycardia syndrome*, Circulation, 2008, - www.ncbi.nlm.nih.gov/pubmed/19808400.

3. For three papers on the Deconditioning Theory

> Levine et al., *Cardiac Origins of the Postural Orthostatic Tachycardia Syndrome*, 2010 - www.ncbi.nlm.nih.gov/pmc/articles/PMC2914315/.
>
> Levine et al., *Effects of exercise training on arterial-cardiac baroreflex function in POTS*, Springer-Verlag, 2011 - http://link.springer.com/article/10.1007%2Fs10286-010-0091-5 (the article can be purchased at this link)
>
> Levine, Shibata, Fu, Bivens, Wang, Hastings., *Short-term exercise training improves the cardiovascular response to exercise in the postural orthostatic tachycardia syndrome*, Journal of Physiology, 2012 - www.ncbi.nlm.nih.gov/pmc/articles/PMC3547265/.

Chapter Two: What is Really Going on in POTS Syndrome & Why it Happens

In chapter one, we considered two of the most important theories for the physiological problems within POTS syndrome. The first concerns the classic signs of deconditioning following a long period of bed rest: POTS patients often have smaller than average hearts and reduced blood volume as a result, both of which lead to the heart having to beat faster in order to compensate for this cardiovascular weakness. The second concerns NET protein deficiency, something which causes simultaneous 'seeping' of adrenalin into the blood stream as well as widening of the blood vessels upon standing when really they should constrict, with the ultimate effect of increased heart rate when orthostatic and a wide range of other symptoms. But which theory points us to the cause? The fundamental deconditioning or the aberrant protein?

To find out the answer we need to look somewhere hitherto unconsidered: the brain. And, in particular, a part of the brain which is utterly essential to nearly every aspect of our lives, namely the 'limbic system', the primitive, yet crucial, mammalian part of our brain, whose job it is to keep us safe, to tell us to fight, freeze or flee, and which connects down into the rest of our body via the entire nervous system. The central claim of this book is that when this part of the brain becomes impaired, for reasons that shall become clear, then it can lead to what we call 'POTS syndrome'. The brain is, in other words, 'the missing link' which can explain the central aspects of pre-existing research into POTS. I note the importance of understanding at this point that I am not - in any way - suggesting POTS syndrome is psychosomatic or 'all in your head', which are ludicrous ideas that a number of POTS patients, before they finally received a correct diagnosis, have had to put up with. Rather, I am discussing a very serious, physical impairment that can occur to the limbic system and the knock-on health effects this impairment can have on the body as a whole. POTS syndrome is a very real *neurological* condition.

In order to state the case for this claim, in this chapter I shall consider, first of all, how the limbic system operates under normal circumstances so as to provide important background information. Then, I shall discuss how the limbic system can, under certain circumstances, enter a state of crisis with direct neurological consequences but also with knock-on consequences on the health of the body. With both of these aspects in place, I shall then consider how these negative changes to the limbic system and knock-on health effects can explain the key findings discussed in the last chapter, thereby showing that limbic system impairment is the 'missing link' in understanding the condition's origins.

The Limbic System Under Normal Circumstances

Before I begin this section, I note here that I owe much of my understanding of the limbic system to Annie Hopper, who works in the field of limbic system dysfunction and rehabilitation, and who herself had a form of limbic system dysfunction called Multiple Chemical Sensitivity (a condition which we shall consider more closely later in the book). I also note that the limbic system is far more complicated than the briefest of sketches I am able to provide here. Rather, my aim in this section is just to focus on the most important functions of the limbic system so that you can best understand later in this chapter how its malfunctioning can lead to POTS syndrome.

How can we best describe the limbic system in a general way? Hopper's description of it as follows is a good place to start. The limbic system is:

"...the part of the brain that is responsible for interpreting, categorizing, and sorting sensory input. It filters the billion bits of information that we experience at any given moment, and determines how we code, remember, and respond to them. It stores memories, regulates hormones, and is also involved in motor function. The limbic system is a large part of our primitive defense mechanism."[23]

Indeed, the word 'limbic' itself comes from the Latin 'limbus', which means 'protection'. It is the part of the

---

[23] Hopper (2014), 13-14.

brain entirely responsible for keeping us safe and for ensuring - in many different ways - that we stay alive. It interprets what we experience and, based on this reading, sends a 'myriad' of signals to the rest of our body.

Let us now consider the function of four crucial parts of the limbic system under normal circumstances: the amygdala, hippocampus, cingulate cortex and hypothalamus.

The amygdala is classically understood as the 'survival' centre of the brain. It is able to send quick protective messages in response to immediate danger. If you have ever unthinkingly walked onto a road only to see a car fast approaching, you don't have to think twice about getting out of the way: your amygdala has sent your body the message to get out of the way without any 'conscious' decision to do so on your part. (Although, sometimes, the amygdala will also send a message to 'freeze' on the spot - note the way animals can 'freeze' in the headlights of oncoming cars at night). The healthy amygdala only senses what danger is present when it *actually* is present. When danger is not present, the fear centres of the amygdala prefer to take a back seat, stay calm and thereby allow the body to be in a peaceful and restorative state.

The hippocampus stores memories. For our purposes, it is important to note that it stores the messages sent out by the amygdala as specific memories, which can be recalled at a later date, when needed. To use a (hopefully) unlikely example, if you have been chased by a tiger and happen to see a real tiger again in the flesh - even if it is behind bars in the zoo - the hippocampus will almost certainly replay the images in your mind of your previous encounter with a tiger. These memories are not accompanied by neutral feelings. A sense of value, importance and meaning is also attached to each memory by the hippocampus. A negative memory of something which caused fear will be stored with 'high importance', and will carry extra weight in your brain. The hippocampus does this for your survival, and it is an essential function. Having said that, when danger is not present, the fear centres in the hippocampus should not be active.

The cingulate cortex is concerned with many of the same aspects as the amygdala and hippocampus, including memory, emotional processing and learning. But it is also, interestingly, concerned with ascertaining how 'safe' stimuli are, both the stimuli from within our own body (e.g. 'Am I too close to the fire?' or 'The pebble in my shoe is hurting my foot!') and sensory stimuli in the external world. Accordingly, it is also the part of the brain particularly associated with processing smell, and in particular smells that are perceived to be dangerous (such as the smell of gas). For example, if you would be unlucky enough to be overexposed to chemicals, your cingulate cortex would fire up into overdrive, sending alarm signals to get away from the noxious smell.

Onto the final - and most important part for understanding POTS syndrome as we shall see - part of the limbic system under discussion, the hypothalamus. For in the hypothalamus we come to see how what is going on in the limbic system really *matters* to the rest of the body. For the hypothalamus' main job is *to take the messages and signals it receives from the other aspects of the limbic system we have just discussed, and repackage them in turn into a collection of messages and signals which the body can understand*. In this way, the hypothalamus is constantly sending out a 'signal' or 'collection of messages' directly to the rest of the body. It does this by sending the signal via the nervous system. As Hopper puts it:

"It (the hypothalamus) is the control center of all autonomic regulatory activities of the body. It is like having an internal chemist as it produces powerful brain hormones which relay information and instructions to all parts of the brain and body. It is responsible for maintaining homeostasis in the body through the cardiovascular system, temperature regulation, and abdominal visceral regulation. It manages endocrine hormonal levels, sensory processing, body metabolism, eating and drinking behaviours."[24]

The signal that the hypothalamus emits is sent via the 'HPA axis', or the 'Hypothalamus-Pituitary-Adrenal Gland Axis' (this can also be understood as the signal the limbic system sends to the entire nervous system). If the signal is one of fear ('flight or fight'), then the signal along the entire nervous system via the HPA axis will instruct the body to prepare for danger. If the signal is one of calm, then the signal the body receives

---

[24] 2014, 18-19.

from the brain will be one of rest and restoration. These two kinds of signal (put here in a very general way) are also referred to as the 'sympathetic branch of the nervous system' (the flight or fight system) and the 'parasympathetic branch of the nervous system' (the rest and digest system). These branches do not act 'of their own accord'. Rather, they act depending on the signal they receive from the limbic system via the HPA axis. Therefore, what is happening in the limbic system is a matter of utmost importance to the body as a whole.

The way I have described the limbic system so far has been very 'top-down', but, crucially, it also works in another way, i.e. 'bottom-up'. For the limbic system does not just emit signals to the nervous system but also *receives* signals, in turn, from the nervous system itself (notice how you can sense the signals from your own body right now in this moment). This is the 'body-mind' connection (as opposed to 'mind-body'). In this way, *what matters to the body also really matters to the brain*. Things work two ways, therefore. This is an absolutely essential point and one which explains why, as we shall see shortly, traumatic illnesses (such as viruses) which affect the body can also affect the limbic system adversely.

Limbic System Malfunction and Disorganisation

So much for the limbic system as it should operate under normal circumstances: what about the possibility of limbic system malfunction?

The limbic system is a vulnerable and sensitive part of the brain, and it is particularly sensitive to events. This is already well-known with the case of PTSD or Post-Traumatic Stress Disorder, where the limbic system becomes damaged as a result of a psychological trauma. PTSD is a very serious kind of limbic system dysfunction and it occurs primarily as a result of a traumatic external experience (although this could also involve internal elements, i.e. if the traumatic event also leads to physical injury such as might occur in a car accident).

But the limbic system is also immensely vulnerable to events that occur in the 'body-mind' connection. For, as I have just mentioned, the limbic system does not just receive our outer experience but also our inner experience and, as such, it is also affected deeply by events that are happening to and in the body. *The main claim that I am making in this regard is that the limbic system can be deeply affected by physical traumas to the body itself.* There are many kinds of physical trauma which the limbic system could register as traumatic, such as:

- an intrusive physical trauma on the body, as in a violent physical assault; a serious surgical operation or a difficult pregnancy [i.e. *limbic system crisis induced by injury*]
- a severe illness which is so severe that, from the brain's point of view, the illness is a 'traumatic event'. Common examples are mononucleosis and Lyme disease, but it could be any severe illness [*i.e. limbic system crisis induced by illness*]

The hardwired state of crisis I am discussing comes about because the limbic system 'reads' - via the 'body-mind' connection - the distress signals ongoing in the body during one of these traumas (such as a severe viral illness) and enters a state of profound crisis as a result. Indeed, depending on the severity of such a 'triggering event', it is biologically possible for the limbic system to enter a state of *hardwired and perpetual* crisis. This state of crisis has far-reaching neurological effects and knock-on effects on the entire body (as we shall see), for, as mentioned above, things work two ways. A distress signal from the body is 'sent up' to the limbic system via the nervous system, affecting the limbic system and changing, in turn, the signal that the limbic system 'sends back down' to the body via the nervous system. Indeed, this complex receiving and emitting of signals is best understood as a kind of 'signal loop'.

If it seems strange or unlikely that the limbic system might be affected by these kinds of events, then there are a few points to consider. In the case of a viral illness, remember that the limbic system is deeply involved, in its protective role, whenever we have an illness. The initial viral illness involves, of course, the virus running its course and during this time our limbic system's survival signals become stronger and highly active as part of an effort to defeat the illness. But say the effects of the viral illness on the body are so severe that, long after the virus itself has left the body, the brain itself remains in a traumatic state as a result of the signals it received during the illness. It remains stuck, in other words, in the 'survival mode' which it was in during the illness itself: *the brain still believes it is necessary to protect the person from the physical difficulties it sensed from the virus*. This is because the 'distress signals' that the body was sending up to the brain during the illness were so severe that the brain redoubled its efforts at protecting the person concerned, and, thanks to neuroplasticity (a concept we shall consider later on and which concerns the brain's ability to change in response to experience), the brain remained 'stuck' in this highly protective mode after the virus had run its course. The brain remained stuck, in other words, in survival mode. Likewise, the effects a difficult pregnancy can have on the brain are not as yet understood, even though it is currently recognised, as Brooks, McCully and Cassaglia write, that pregnancy '...increases sympathetic nerve firing and decreases...parasympathetic activity'.[25] In such a case, the difficulties of the pregnancy could also leave the brain stuck in a traumatic, self-protective state. Culturally speaking we tend to be myopic about the full range of ways that the limbic system can be affected by events, only really aware of the ways in which the limbic system can be affected by psychological events (as in the case of PTSD). Biologically speaking, however, it stands to reason that distress signals emitted via the nervous system to the limbic system during a severe illness could act as a kind of 'internal trigger' that would also force the limbic system to enter a state of perpetual crisis.

---

[25] *ANS Primer*, chapter 55, 2015.

In emphasising these 'physical' traumatic triggers, however, I am not discounting the role that psychological traumas may play in the development of limbic system impairment. However, in these cases, as with PTSD, the person concerned also has no 'choice' in the matter. For, at a psychological level also, the limbic system operates in automatic and primitive ways. It experiences an event and the chemical response it creates as a result happens with no conscious effort on the part of the individual: it is all automatic. No one, indeed, would choose to have PTSD. The war veteran who experiences constant flashbacks does not 'choose' to do so: rather his or her limbic system entered a state of hyper-vigilant crisis *automatically* in response to the experiences of the horrors of war. The rational part of their mind knows that the original traumatic danger is no longer present but the limbic system has remained stuck in a traumatic state thanks to a maladaptive and automatic neuroplastic response. In any event, the point is that it is possible that psychological traumas - whether on their own or in addition to physical traumas - may contribute to the development of limbic system impairment too. Having made these distinctions, however, I also note that the distinctions between 'physical' and 'psychological' trauma can also break down quite easily. Every trauma has both physical and psychological components, although it is helpful to categorise some as being more physical than psychological and vice versa. Of course, psychological and physical limbic system traumas might also combine, creating a 'perfect storm' of trauma. Similarly, traumas do not always need to be acute, relating to one specific incident in time. Rather there could be a series of traumas over several years, each one leading to a more hyper-sensitive limbic system, with a final trauma occurring as the catalyst for a state of total limbic system trauma.

In general, is not so important how the limbic system enters a state of crisis more than the fact that it does so. Whatever the nature of the trigger, however, it is essential to remember that the person affected has had no say in the matter. The limbic system responds to events in automatic ways and according to its own primitive biological laws - whether that trauma was more physical or more psychological. For these reasons, I refer to any trauma that is capable of tipping the limbic system into crisis as a trauma 'broadly understood'. This includes the possibility of the traumatic trigger being psychological, physical or a combination of both. It also includes the possibility of it being sudden and acute or insidious and building up over a longer period of time.

The Anatomy of the Limbic System in Crisis: What Changes Actually Take Place

The brain is highly 'neuroplastic', that is to say its structure is highly malleable or changeable, especially in response to experience. (We shall consider the science of 'neuroplasticity' in more detail in chapter four). The way in which the brain responds to trauma is no exception. Let us now consider how the limbic system can change in response to the kind of traumatic or 'triggering' events discussed in the last section, including physical traumas (such as a viral illness), crushing psychological traumas, or a combination.

Upon the occurrence of the initial trauma (broadly understood), the distress signals (either internal or external) cause the normal limbic system's neuronal circuits to be broken apart aggressively and disorganised. In this way, the old generally 'calm' neuronal programming in the limbic system is replaced by new, highly fearful brain circuitry which see their job to be the avoidance of any further threat. This highly self-protective neuronal circuitry becomes ever more self-protective and ever more sensitive as time goes on.

The effects of limbic system trauma can be divided into two categories: direct neurological effects and knock-on effects on the health of the body.

To consider the direct neurological effects first, what can primarily be observed is damage to the limbic system's role in perceiving stimuli - both internal and external. Thus, the more the limbic system enters a crisis state, the more likely it is that common stimuli will also begin to be perceived as 'too much'. Loud sounds startle, bright light can give migraines and the scent of chemicals is suddenly perceived by the brain as more powerful than before or even as noxious. The sense of smell of a person with limbic system impairment can actually change drastically (interestingly the limbic system used to be referred to as the 'rhinocephalon' or 'centre of the nose', given its role in processing smell). As time goes by and the brain becomes more and more hypervigilant, it is possible for this sensitivity to become extreme. For example, it may be impossible to tolerate light at all. Chemical exposure may lead to anaphylactic shock. It is even possible to develop sensitivity to electro-magnetic frequencies. Similarly, the perception of internal stimuli can also go wrong. In particular, the pain centres of the limbic system become overly active, leading to perceiving pain and tenderness in all aspects of the body. These direct neurological changes as a result of a trauma to the limbic system lead to a kind of ongoing neurological nightmare.

However, these direct neurological changes also lead to knock-on effects on the health of the body. This is because of the role of the hypothalamus in sending a 'signal' to the entire nervous system via the HPA axis. How the nervous system behaves depends entirely upon the 'quality' of this signal. When the limbic system is in crisis, the HPA axis is constantly 'firing off' and constantly sending out messages for adrenalin to be released. The result is that the parasympathetic nervous system (the rest and digest system) is no longer given permission to do the work it needs to do, with widespread disastrous results. Energy production falls, the body is unable to receive nourishment as a result of impaired digestion, the thyroid suffers as do the hormone, immune and endocrine systems. Hopper describes the vicious cycle that ensues as follows:

"A limbic system impairment is psychoneuroimmunological (PNI) in nature, which means it involves psychological processes as well as the nervous and immune systems of the body....the brain gets 'stuck' in an unconscious state of chronic emergency that perpetuates illness and inflammation. This typically involves the central nervous system, the musculoskeletal system, and the endocrine system."[26]

A limbic system impairment really is a two-fold problem, therefore. The sufferer must contend with the direct neurological effects of the crisis as well as the knock-on effects on the health of the body as a result of the compromised nervous system as a whole. The problem, however, is that medical research into what are in fact limbic system impairments has tended to miss the root cause, focussing instead on treating the secondary, 'knock-on' health effects on the body and on assuming that the root cause of the condition will be found amongst these secondary effects. This is the equivalent of studying a tree's branches for signs of disease when actually the tree's problems may actually be located in its roots.

Summary of a Limbic System in Crisis

In conclusion to this section, you need to remember the following four points:

i) the brain, especially the limbic system, is very vulnerable to experience and its structure changes in response to life's events. This is particularly true of traumatic events, where 'traumatic' is understood broadly to include physical traumas (such as a virus or pregnancy), crushing psychological traumas or a combination.

---

[26] 2014, 22.

ii) The limbic system enters a resulting hardwired state of crisis either via the body-mind or mind-body connection (or both) and this can cause widespread negative (and hardwired) structural changes in the brain.

iii) The first kind of adverse effect of this change concerns the limbic system's ability to perceive stimuli: the faculties of sound, light, and smell are all adversely affected and become hypervigilant, sometimes extremely so.

iv) The second effect of limbic system impairment is on the body. When the limbic system is in crisis, the HPA axis is constantly emitting a crisis signal, which leads the nervous system, in turn, to malfunction, with the sympathetic branch dominating, leading to widespread changes in energy production, the endocrine and hormonal systems and many others essential aspects of the body's health.

These are serious neurological changes even if they are not, as yet, the subject of the serious neurological study they deserve. In fact, despite the study of the limbic system in medical school, it is often assumed that its disorders must necessarily belong to the realm of psychology. This is a tragic mistake as it ignores both the role the limbic system, through its connection to the nervous system, necessarily plays in overall health and the fact that 'non-psychological' events can adversely impact limbic system function through the 'body-mind' connection. As a result, many with limbic system impairment who present to their doctor will find that their myriad of symptoms are treated individually, as if each symptom were happening of 'its own accord', rather than receiving a treatment plan for the root cause of all the symptoms. Worse is the fact that some medical professionals, given the intense anxiety patients with limbic system trauma often understandably feel, will dismiss these patients as suffering from psychosomatic complaints, rather than a genuine brain-malfunction, the development of which the individual had no say in. Indeed, I will have more to say countering any suggestion that limbic system impairment is 'psychosomatic' at the end of this chapter.

What POTS Syndrome Really Is

We are now in a position to come to the crux of this book: to understand what POTS syndrome really is. Be prepared to change what you thought you knew about POTS: it is not primarily a cardiac problem, the result of being unfit, or the inability of the body (somehow or other) to deal with the effects of gravity, as is sometimes suggested.

Here we go:

POTS Syndrome is a Form of Limbic System Dysfunction.

In other words, *POTS syndrome is caused by a limbic system in crisis along with the knock-on adverse effects on the body that involves, following a traumatic event, broadly understood to include physical traumas (such as a viral illness) or psychological traumas (or both).*

And now I'm going to attempt to spell out exactly *how*.

Explaining POTS Syndrome: What is Really Going On

In chapter one, I discussed the two 'schools of thought' on the origins of POTS syndrome, the 'deconditioning argument' and the 'NET protein' deficiency argument. I will state my position on both right now, and then expand: deconditioning is not the cause of POTS, although it does play a secondary role. The NET, or Norepinephrine Reuptake Transporter protein, hypothesis, however, is the one which points to the true origins of POTS, and it is the key pre-existing finding in medical research into the condition which can be explained as a direct result of limbic system impairment.

Why?

There are three reasons:

i) The cause of NET deficiency has been shown not to be genetic, therefore it must be caused by some *other* reason. NET cannot become deficient just 'because it feels like it'.

ii) Norepinephrine and Adrenalin are the same substance.

iii) When the Limbic system is in crisis, the HPA axis is always active and adrenalin is being released nearly *all the time*.

Taking these three points, I will now explain by using an example how the limbic system in crisis leads to NET deficiency.

The POTS patient suffers from some kind of 'traumatic' event (broadly understood), such as a viral illness, surgery or difficult pregnancy. Long after this event has occurred, the brain of the POTS patient remains 'stuck' in limbic system trauma thanks to a maladaptive neuroplastic response to that trauma. This response came about as a result of intense distress signals the brain received during that trauma. The patient's brain thus enters a highly self-protective state: sensory perception changes and the patient becomes sensitive to light, sound and smell. The HPA axis works overtime, sending alarm messages to the adrenal glands which, in turn, send out adrenalin all the time. If you are a POTS patient, consider right now whether the feeling of adrenalin regularly 'firing off' is a familiar one to you. This is evidence that the origin of the problem is neurological.

Now, for quite some time, the NET protein just about manages to deal with the job of recycling all this excess adrenalin. After all, that's what it has been designed to do. When adrenalin is in the blood stream, NET gets on with storing and recycling it. But what about when there is simply too much of the hormone around? What happens to the NET protein when it becomes 'overwhelmed'?

My main thesis is that at a certain point NET *becomes no longer able to cope*: it breaks down and ceases to work properly. In much the same way that a fatigued muscle has a 'breaking point' beyond which it can no longer do its work, so too does NET have a 'breaking point' after which it can no longer deal with its primary task of recycling adrenalin. There has simply been too much of the hormone and for too long. Once it breaks down, the NET protein has become *deficient*. It is no longer 'strong enough' to do its job and keep blood vessels constricted in the way they should be upon standing. Likewise, it is no longer 'strong enough' to recycle all of the adrenalin it should be able to recycle. The result, as we have seen in chapter one, is twofold: that *the blood vessels remain wider than they should be upon standing and the heart must beat faster to compensate so as to maintain blood flow over a larger area* and, secondly, *that more and more adrenalin spills out into the blood stream and makes contact with the heart, causing it to beat faster still*. You cannot hold the plank position forever and, likewise, the NET protein, although it has been designed to recycle and make use of adrenalin, will reach a point where there is too much adrenalin 'washing over it' for it to be able to perform this task. In short: the NET protein is primed to transport and recycle all available adrenalin but when there is a huge amount of that hormone available *all the time*, the NET protein eventually becomes exhausted and unable to function properly.

In making this connection between the limbic system in crisis and the malfunctioning of the NET protein, I am trying to 'connect the dots'. If NET is deficient in POTS patients, and we know that it is, and if this is not the result of genetics, which we also know that it is not, then, surely, the only adequate explanation is that NET has become deficient through the excess supply of adrenalin, and that the root cause of this can only be found in the brain, and in particular the limbic system? I cannot see any other reason for NET having become deficient. It cannot, for example, become deficient through cardiovascular weakness (for in that case most of the elderly would have NET deficiency). For the same reasons, I cannot see any other reason why the POTS patient should be 'hyperadrenergic', other than the limbic system entering continuous crisis along with the frequent release of adrenalin which that entails.

Furthermore, this theory I am putting forward takes very seriously the idea that POTS is preceded by a triggering event. You will remember in chapter one that I outlined the mainstream view that POTS nearly always is preceded by a triggering event, but that the connection between such an event and the onset of the condition has not been studied. Nevertheless, it seems to be a constant that can be observed and as such it *must* hold the key to the condition. It is rare, if you read a story about how someone developed POTS in the media for example, that you do not also read of some kind of antecedent illness. There must be a reason why this is the case. I believe that it is because the antecedent illness is so severe that the distress signals the body emits to the brain during the course of that illness force the limbic system to enter a state of hardwired neurological crisis. Furthermore, it should be noted that all kinds of antecedent illnesses seem to lead to POTS syndrome. I have used mononucleosis and

Lyme disease as my main examples but one reads of many different preceding illnesses from bacterial infections to salmonella poisoning. The fact that there are a variety of possible 'triggering' illnesses shows that their significance is to be found in the *severity* of the illnesses in question: that is their common link. In other words, it would be misguided to think that there may be something specific in mononucleosis (rather than Lyme disease, say) that holds the key to understanding POTS or vice versa. Rather the key thing is that both illnesses - and all others which trigger POTS - tend to be *severe*. It is this severity which explains why the brain is adversely impacted by such illnesses.

I hope that this chapter will have shown that the fact that there is a triggering event is not merely a side point, *but the key to the whole condition and something which illustrates that the condition clearly stems from a brain impairment.*

Conclusions I: From POTS to LSIND

In summary, POTS Syndrome could be better defined as the following:

"A state of hard-wired "trauma" in the limbic system from a triggering event where trauma is understood broadly to include physical traumas such as a viral illness. This state of hardwired trauma leads to the release of continuous crisis signals via the HPA axis (including the frequent release of adrenalin) which leads, in turn, to NET deficiency along with deficient vasoconstriction, a hyperadrenergic state, and resulting tachycardia as a result of this deficient vasoconstricion and increased adrenalin. This limbic system dysfunction also leads to a wide range of problems in the nervous system, affecting digestion, the hormonal and endocrine systems, energy production and sensory perception in the limbic system, with increased sensitivity to light, sound and smell."

In other words, POTS is not primarily a cardiac problem: it is a neurological one with widespread effects on the entire body. Given this, what should the condition really be called? I would suggest that a more accurate name might be LSIND or *'Limbic System Induced NET Deficiency'*, as that covers the key neurological and cardiovascular problems in the condition, and the relation of the one to the other.

There are, of course, advantages to using the term 'POTS' to describe the condition, primarily because this term has now been used for quite some time and considerable awareness has been raised about the condition. In other ways, however, POTS is an unhelpful term in that many do not grasp the significance of the 'S' or 'Syndrome' part of the acronym, and actually *define* the condition as being a problem with 'dealing with gravity'. I believe that calling this condition 'POTS' has meant that its seriousness has not been fully grasped. It is easier not to grasp the severity of the condition if it merely seems to involve problems standing up, a fact that has led some to call it merely a 'nuisance' condition (although I would challenge anyone who says this to stand by the idea that being unable to stand up without difficulty is merely a 'nuisance'!). There is another problem with the term 'POTS' in that it places too much emphasis on the idea that the condition is primarily postural. Now, of course, as we know, the patient is indeed particularly affected upon standing up for that is when the NET protein must do its primary work. But that is just a side-effect of the actual root cause of the condition, which is a form of neurological impairment. Indeed, although it is essential that the POTS patient understands the difficulties she will face upon standing, it is misleading to define the condition as being a problem *with* standing up. After all, if the theory I am putting forward is true, this is happening only as a knock-on effect of an ongoing neurological crisis.

I note that the other term used for the condition, 'dysautonomia' is undoubtedly more accurate than POTS. However, it too gives a somewhat false impression. Why? *It leaves out the limbic system, which is the root of the nervous system*. Indeed, it gives the impression that the nervous system has gone into crisis "of its own accord". To the patient, 'dysautonomia' has a cruel finality to it: *my nervous system has gone haywire and there is nothing I can do about it*. This description ignores, however, the scientific fact that the nervous system takes its 'cue' for how to behave from the 'signal' it constantly receives from the limbic system: it does not act "of its own accord" and it certainly does not go into crisis for reasons known only to itself.

Conclusions II: POTS is Caused by the Brain But it is Not Psychosomatic

It should be obvious from the discussion in this chapter that to say POTS is caused by limbic system impairment is not to suggest that it is psychosomatic. A psychosomatic illness has negative (and often deeply misguided and prejudiced) connotations attached to the term which suggest that some people can 'think themselves into' a state of illness. Leaving aside the question of whether this is even biologically possible, it certainly does not apply to POTS syndrome. Rather, something overwhelmingly terrible happens, such as a viral illness, and the limbic system perceives this to be so threatening to the organism's survival that it rewires itself of its own accord into a hard-wired protective and crisis state. The limbic system is a primitive part of the brain and it does this in automatic ways which the individual concerned has no say in. Even if the initial trigger is a psychological one, as can be the case, the individual has no say in this either as the limbic system also acts automatically and of its own accord in these cases too (as is the way in PTSD also). So there should never be any fault or blame imputed onto the patient with POTS. In the same way that a war veteran with PTSD should never be 'blamed' for how his or her primitive limbic system reacted to the horrors of war, so too should a POTS patient not be blamed for how his or her primitive limbic system reacted to an antecedent 'triggering' traumatic illness or other trauma.

Indeed, I believe that there is an understandable fear amongst patients and medical researchers alike that the condition might ever appear to be 'psychosomatic'. This is understandable as a) it is plain wrong to regard POTS as such and b) it would falsely stigmatise those suffering with this devastating condition. However, the efforts to avoid the psychosomatic label may have led POTS research away from where it needs to go. For example, the fact that there is extra sympathetic discharge in POTS patients appears to be well-known but there has been - perhaps - an unwillingness to consider the role of the brain in emitting this extra sympathetic discharge because that might appear - on the face of it - to imply that POTS is a psychological problem, no different from an anxiety disorder. Instead, research has focussed on NET deficiency as being the key reason for the extra adrenalin that exists in the POTS patient's blood stream, not realising that NET has probably become deficient in the first place because the brain is in crisis. Whilst this fear is understandable, I hope I have shown it is also misguided. For the limbic system in the case of POTS is not the same as the limbic system in a state of (psychological) anxiety. There is more than one way for a limbic system to enter a crisis, and the limbic system is not just affected by psychological traumas, as I have pointed out, but also by the body-mind connection and the kind of 'distress' signals the limbic system can receive during a severe illness. If the significance of this could be grasped then I think there would not need to be any fear of the condition ever being falsely labelled as 'psychosomatic'. Furthermore, it needs to be remembered that the limbic system is primitive and responds automatically to events following its own laws such that even in the case of crushing psychological triggers, these too are not the 'fault' of the individual concerned. However, we are culturally myopic about both of these aspects. As regards the former, we have little awareness of how the brain can be affected by signals coming from the body and, as regards the latter, many - almost always those who have not experienced a trauma themselves - do not understand the ways in which the brain can be affected by events. For example, it's easy for the person without PTSD to tell someone who has it to 'snap out of it', but that person simply has no idea what suffering with a limbic system impairment is like. For when the limbic system is calm, you don't notice its workings. When it is in crisis, however, its immense power and huge role in our overall physical and psychological health become overwhelmingly apparent.

Key Points of Chapter Two

In this chapter, I have set out the theory that it is possible for the limbic system to enter a perpetual crisis state following an initial trauma, broadly understood. I have put forward an hypothesis as to how this perpetual crisis state can explain the core findings of those with POTS syndrome: a hyperadrenergic state and NET deficiency. The limbic system in crisis leads to the constant release of adrenalin which, in time, leads the NET protein to break down. You cannot do push ups for ever and nor can the NET protein do its job forever of recycling available adrenalin. Based on this, I suggest the condition might instead be more accurately termed LSIND: 'Limbic System Induced NET Deficiency' and that any reference to it as 'dysautonomia' should also recognise the role of the limbic system in the autonomic nervous system.

Further Reading

Hopper, A., *Wired for Healing: Remapping the Brain to Recover From Chronic and Mysterious Illnesses*, Friesens, 2014.

Chapter Three: Explaining the Whole Elephant (or How Limbic System Malfunction Can Explain Everything We Know About POTS)

In the introduction, we first considered the elephant analogy used by Prof. Satish Raj, a researcher on POTS at the University of Calgary. Several blind men are each holding different parts of an elephant. As they only focus on *parts* of the elephant however, they cannot grasp the *whole* of the creature, and so they do not realise that they are, in fact, holding parts of an elephant: they make incorrect guesses as they are unable to see the big picture. I believe this analogy holds true. In this chapter, I will suggest how understanding the condition as a limbic system impairment could arguably explain all the various so-called 'POTS sub-types' or how, in other words, understanding the neurological origins of POTS can explain the 'whole elephant'. Furthermore, the idea of limbic system impairment can also potentially explain other overlapping conditions that the POTS patient often has, such as chronic fatigue syndrome (M.E.) and fibromyalgia. Having said that, the explanation of NET deficiency as having been caused by a limbic system impairment remains this book's most important potential contribution as NET deficiency is the principal reason the POTS patient's heart rate increases upon standing up (as a result of vasoconstriction deficiency).

The Misplaced Idea of POTS 'Subtypes'

In my view, it is a mistake to hold too rigidly to the idea that there are separate kinds of POTS, or 'POTS subtypes'. The usual story of POTS subtypes goes something like this: you have either the 'hyperadrenergic' form of POTS, the 'deconditioning' form, or the 'neuropathic' form. In addition, there are also other potential subtypes: the POTS which co-exists with viral antibodies, or the POTS which is caused by having defective collagen production (as found in Ehlers-Danlos Syndrome or Joint Hypermobility Syndrome), or the type of POTS which is defined by the co-existence of mast cell activation problems. However, I would argue that this tendency to try to place POTS into more manageable 'subtypes' is misguided and the equivalent of the blind men being unable to see the elephant before them. Indeed, the 'breaking up' of POTS into little pieces is part of the problem, not the solution. As Raj writes: 'These subtypes may be of value in trying to understand the pathophysiology of POTS, and may help to develop rational therapeutic approaches. However, it is currently quite difficult to characterize an individual patient as belonging to one particular subtype. The putative pathophysiological mechanisms...are not mutually exclusive, and can co-exist in a particular individual.'[27] As these so-called

---

[27] *ANS Primer*, chapter 107.

subtypes can indeed co-exist in any given individual, then what if there were a root cause which could explain *all* of them? Let's see if the limbic system hypothesis might be able to. In addition, I will also attempt to put forward suggestions as to how the limbic system impairment hypothesis could potentially explain disturbances in the renin-angiotensin-aldosterone network, a key factor in low blood volume in POTS.

Explaining the POTS Elephant: There are no 'POTS Subtypes' Just Limbic System Dysfunction which Affects the Body in Different Ways

i) *'Hyperadrenergic POTS'*

There is little which needs to be said about the hyperadrenergic 'subtype' as it was the subject of the last chapter. Many POTS patients have high levels of adrenalin in their blood stream for reasons we have already seen, as the level of norepinephrine in the blood depends on the state of the NET protein. The amount of adrenalin in the blood stream varies depending on the extent of this deficiency (and the extent of the crisis in the brain).

ii) *'Deconditioned POTS'*

I will consider the deconditioning theory in more detail than the other subtypes, as it is one of the more prevalent hypotheses on the origin of POTS. I would argue that, whilst it is true that deconditioning necessarily plays a considerable role in POTS patients, and that research into it is *very* important (for it shows that cardiovascular reconditioning will necessarily be an important part of making a full recovery), deconditioning itself is not the cause of POTS, but rather an additional consequence of limbic system induced NET deficiency. It is the latter, the inability of blood vessels to constrict upon standing, which leads to the patient having such difficulty with any physical tasks with the result that they become deconditioned. The simple fact is this: *if you have POTS for any substantial length of time, you will become deconditioned.* In the 2012 Levine study on the effects of cardiovascular exercise on POTS patients, the patients in the study had had the condition at the least for six months before participation and, at the most, for five years. If you are hardly able to do any physical activity for such lengths of time, *you will become very unfit.* In that sense, it is absolutely correct to say that a period of bed rest can lead to extreme cardiovascular deconditioning, and that any treatment protocol for POTS must take into account the severity of those effects and the importance of treating them through exercise.

There are, however, several further arguments from common sense against considering deconditioning as the root cause of POTS.

Firstly, if it were true, then POTS would be an extremely prevalent condition. It would be common for the elderly to develop POTS. This is not the case. Instead, an unlucky (if sizeable) minority have it, among them children, teenagers and young adults - many of whom were fit and well before the condition's onset. How could a ten-year-old child possibly be *so* deconditioned as to develop POTS whilst an elderly person who has not moved much for several decades does not develop it? The argument that a period of bed rest causes POTS is also surely misguided (even though prolonged bed rest undoubtedly *does* cause cardiac deconditioning). The overwhelming majority of people who have enforced periods of bed rest do not develop the symptoms of POTS (even though they become weak). Similarly, many who have been disabled for other reasons - such as through paralysis or loss of limb - also do not develop the symptoms of POTS despite being unable to do any activity whatsoever for decades.

Secondly, if deconditioning really were the cause, then, after say six months intensive cardiovascular training, it should be possible to cease this intensive exercise, and instead engage in basic cardiovascular work. Once the deconditioned person has become 'reconditioned', they should be *cured*. But, in practice, this is not what seems to happen: the patient has to keep up the cardiovascular work at a high intensity for as long as they live. This cannot be right. Rather, their symptoms have been ameliorated, by having increased blood volume through having a stronger heart. As a result, their system is better able to cope with the limbic system dysfunction and resultant NET deficiency, but that, I would suggest, is all. In this way, cardiovascular exercise is the physical equivalent of taking more salt and liquid to boost blood volume. It really helps, but it does not fix the cause. The main point is this: a cure should result in the supine-to-standing differential returning to normal, i.e. a 10-20 beats increase upon standing. It seems that this is not generally what seems to happen to those following the cardiovascular retraining programs: their differential remains higher than that as does their standing heart rate.

The research into deconditioning in POTS, however, is ultimately helpful, in that it shows the importance of cardiovascular reconditioning as an important addition to treatment. However, the problem - in terms of grasping the overall complexity of POTS - is that the deconditioning theory is sometimes presented as being 'the' root cause. In a 2011 study, Levine et al., wrote that POTS:

"...patients have often been described as having a "dysautonomia". However investigations regarding the function of the autonomic nervous system in patients with POTS have not been extensive, with controversial results...We recently found that POTS patients, as a group, had normal autonomic function, while the marked tachycardia during orthostasis appeared to be a physiological compensatory response to a small stroke volume which was attributable to a small heart coupled with reduced blood volume...These results suggest that POTS per se is a consequence of "deconditioning"."[28]

---

[28] 74.

I note that this claim was made before the dysfunction of the NET protein was established as being a certainty in the POTS patient through other research, and it might well be the case that Levine at al., would no longer be of this view. Indeed, the autonomic nervous system tests they ran did not appear to include either tests for hyperadrenergism or NET deficiency. In any event, I hope that one day deconditioning in POTS will be seen for what it is: one factor of many in understanding the 'whole elephant' of POTS and what is required to treat the after-effects of the condition but *not* something which is the reason for the 'elephant' itself.

iii) Renin-Angiotensin-Aldosterone Problems in POTS Patients (and resulting low blood volume / hypovolemia)

Another problem often identified in POTS patients is to be found in the Renin-Angiotensin-Aldosterone (RAA) axis. The actions of this axis are complex. Suffice to say that the correct functioning of this axis is important for maintaining adequate blood volume, the balance of various electrolytes in the blood, and a balanced endocrine system. It has been found that POTS patients often have low levels of renin and aldosterone in their blood stream. One of the functions of both of these substances is to hold onto the body's salt supply. When both of these are at low levels, the body's ability to hold onto salt (sodium) is accordingly impaired. It is known that the inability of the body to hold onto salt can lead to low blood volume, as salt raises blood volume. This is an essential point as it is well-known that low-blood volume (hypovolemia) contributes to POTS patients' symptoms significantly. As Raj writes: 'These data suggest that abnormalities in the renin-angiotensin-aldosterone axis might have a role in the pathophysiology of POTS by contributing to hypovolemia (low blood volume) and impaired sodium retention.'[29] It is because of low aldosterone levels in POTS patients that they are often given a drug called 'Flurinef' which is a synthetic form of aldosterone, so as to boost the levels of aldosterone and thereby increase blood volume. Similarly, POTS patients are usually advised to 'salt load' their diets to address their poor sodium retention mechanisms as a result of the low aldosterone and renin.

It might seem that problems with low renin and aldosterone levels are an example of the body 'just not working properly', and that the only way to aid the situation is through drugs which ramp up the levels of these substances. But a limbic system in crisis can, again, potentially explain what is really going on with the renin-angiotensin-aldosterone network. For aldosterone is, in fact, *secreted from the adrenal gland*.[30] Now, if that adrenal gland has been overworked to an unbearable level by being forced to release adrenalin continuously, would it not therefore be less able, logically speaking, to produce adequate amounts of aldosterone? Yes, of course. Push something past its breaking point and it can no longer

---

[29] *ANS Primer*, chapter 107.

[30] *ANS Primer*, chapter 23.

function properly. Therefore, we immediately see a reason for the fact that there is less aldosterone in the POTS patient than in the healthy person, which thereby explains the resulting low blood volume through poor sodium retention on that count (for poor sodium retention is a direct result of low aldosterone levels). This aspect of hypovolemia in the POTS patient, therefore, might also result from a limbic system in crisis.

But the limbic system link does not stop there. For the entire renin-angiotensin-aldosterone axis also depends for its own functions completely on the state of the autonomic nervous system. As Pratt writes, the RAA axis '...interacts with the autonomic nervous system for blood pressure regulation, with angiotensin receptors localized to brain regions involved in modulation of both sympathetic and parasympathetic nervous system activity.'[31] In other words, this axis, like the HPA axis, will also go into overdrive when the sympathetic branch of the nervous system is overactive. Indeed, when angiotensin receptors in the brain become active during sympathetic activity, they: '...increase blood pressure, vasoconstriction' and are 'pro-inflammation, pro-oxidative, pro-thirst', and have a role in 'anxiety, stress, neuronal excitation' and 'stimulate aldosterone, norepinephrine...release'.[32] The same old story, in other words. Eventually, the chronic over-activity of the RAA axis will also lead to its malfunction, resulting in low renin and aldosterone levels on that count too.

---

[31] *ANS Primer*, chapter 23.

[32] *ANS Primer*, chapter 23.

For it too takes its 'cue' for how to behave from the signal the limbic system emits.

In short, this malfunctioning of the RAA axis can also be explained by the fact it becomes 'overworked' as a result of taking its 'cue' of how to act from a limbic system in crisis. This, in turn, explains to a large extent the low blood volume (hypovolemia) present in many POTS patients, a factor which is not, therefore, due to deconditioning alone, although deconditioning will also explain hypovolemia to a considerable extent.

iv) *Mast Cell Activation Subtype*

A subset of POTS patients also present with MCAS or 'Mast Cell Activation Syndrome' (this is distinct from MCAD, 'Mast Cell Activation Disorder', which is a genetic disease). Mast cells are a type of white blood cell important in the allergic response. They are responsible for the release of histamine (you may be familiar with the idea that many who suffer with allergies take 'anti-histamine' tablets). When you are stung by a bee, for example, your body releases histamine at the site of the sting. As Raj notes, however, in some patients with POTS, mast cells are likely to be released frequently and for no particularly obvious reason. The symptoms usually involve 'flushing', as well as, as Raj writes 'shortness of breath, headache, light-headedness, excessive diuresis, and gastrointestinal symptoms such as diarrhoea, nausea, and vomiting.'[33] Triggers include, as Raj goes on to say,

---

[33] Raj, 2013.

'...long-term standing, exercise, premenstrual cycle, meals, and sexual intercourse.' The exact reasons for mast cell hyperactivity in POTS patients are currently unknown, although Raj does wonder '...if sympathetic activation, through release of norepineprhine...is the cause of mast cell activation'.

This is undoubtedly correct. For, if the limbic system is in crisis, we know that the body is in crisis, and that adrenalin is, put bluntly, everywhere. In this case, more and more things - previously considered benign by the brain - begin to be perceived as 'dangerous'. It is entirely plausible that, in this way, the signal for mast cells to release histamine is also overactive and that the 'triggers' required for this activation become increasingly 'trivial'. For example, certain foods may start to be detected by the brain and body as 'dangerous', leading to the release of histamine after a meal. The 'crisis state' in the brain can lead to the creation of all kinds of allergies one would not have otherwise. Indeed, as with the RAA considered above, the release of histamine is very much related to the sympathetic branch of the nervous system. Lipton describes histamine as 'a local emergency alarm'[34]: histamine is all about *protection in response to perceived attack*. Now, if the body and brain are stuck in a constant state of 'perceived attack', why would not mast cell activity also go haywire? It stands to reason that it would.

---

[34] *The Biology of Belief*, 2008, 106.

v) *'Neuropathic' POTS Subtype*

Although I argue that all supposed subtypes of POTS, in fact, overlap, it is currently thought that some patients *primarily* have 'neuropathic POTS'. In practice, this means that a fraction of POTS patients have 'denervation of sympathetic nerves...(in)...the lower limbs'.[35] This means in turn that some patients with POTS have '...less norepinephrine release (less sympathetic activation) in their lower extremities'.[36]

I admit that I am unsure of the exact connection between limbic system dysfunction and this 'subtype', although, on a personal note, I think I remember what it feels like to have this problem (in terms of the 'shooting pains' I experienced in the feet, which are a common symptom of this kind of neuropathy). I wonder, however, if the answer to why this happens might be somewhat simpler than one might guess. We know that in those patients with 'neuropathic POTS', norepinephrine release is '...intact in blood drawn from arm veins but reduced from corresponding leg veins'.[37] In other words, the problem lies in the extremities. Now, could this not be a result of being unable to stand for a while or, at the least, spending most of one's life supine or sitting down (as the more severe kinds of POTS necessitate)? In such cases, there has been far less *circulation* to the extremities, which often become cold (indeed, 'Reynaud's phenomenon', which involves

---

[35] Raj, 2013.

[36] Raj, 2013.

[37] *ANS Primer*, chapter 106.

extremely cold feet and hands, is common in POTS patients). This in itself tells us that there is *not much activity in general* going on in the feet, let alone in their nerves: could this reduced blood flow not impact in some adverse way upon the sympathetic nerves in the extremities? In addition, when the brain is in a crisis state, it looks to preserve what is most vital to its survival, and those are the parts of the body closer to the heart. The feet are not vital under such circumstances, as far as the brain is concerned. Its energies are taken inwards to its most vital functions. This might also explain in some way the partial denervation of the feet. In short, my hunch is that this denervation comes about because, in the more severe cases of POTS, the feet are rarely used and, as such, their normal functions (including nerve function) break down to an extent, and also because the brain in crisis prioritises parts of the body which are more vital (and, in this case, the feet also 'lose out'). If this is correct, then partial denervation in the extremities is not a 'cause' or 'distinct type' of POTS, but merely another consequence of the initial limbic system crisis state. However, these are just suggestions and the actual link between the neuropathic problems identified in POTS and limbic system malfunction remains to be established.

Two Unlikely Causes of POTS

In addition to the five possible 'subsets' of POTS just discussed, I should also add here two other possible 'causes' for POTS which are unlikely to be causal, even though they can co-exist with the condition.

vi) *Antibodies*

The idea that viral antibodies themselves might be a factor in the origins of POTS syndrome is unlikely although, as already explained, a virus may 'trigger' the condition. An antibody is a blood protein produced as part of a 'counteracting response' to a specific antigen. It is a protein which can bind with substances perceived as alien to the body, including viruses, and it can remain in the blood stream. If evidence of the presence of viral antibodies in POTS patients could be proved consistently, it could indicate a possible cause, illustrating the 'after-effects' of the virus. However, this has not been the case. A Mayo clinic trial found only a 7-14% prevalence of a viral antibody in POTS patients. Vanderbilt found *none* over several years of searching.[38] The idea that antibodies might *cause* POTS is therefore extremely unlikely. What is more likely is that some patients, for whatever reason, also develop viral antibodies following infection *separately* to malfunction of their limbic system. Why a small fraction of some patients have antibodies and others do not is unclear. It is equally possible, of course, that someone might have viral antibodies but not have a limbic system in crisis. Therefore, one should not read

---

[38] For both studies, see the Raj lecture ('Connecting the Dots Between EDS and POTS') on YouTube
(www.YouTube.com/watch?v=srUJRRihvsE), at 39.40 and ff.

too much into the antibody theory, the evidence for which is immensely slight in any event.

vii) *Ehlers-Danlos Syndrome (EDS) / Joint Hypermobility Syndrome (JHS)*

EDS or JHS are sometimes suggested as a 'cause' for POTS syndrome in those patients who also have those conditions. EDS is a genetic condition which involves malfunction in the production of collagen - the connective tissue which runs throughout the body and which is responsible for placing limits on how much your skin can be stretched. The collagen malfunction problems in those with EDS mean that their skin in particular tends, accordingly, to be stretched very easily. Furthermore, those with EDS tend to be very "hyper-mobile": their joints can easily dislocate and many parts of their body are overtly flexible. JHS involves the same hyper-flexibility, although usually to a lesser extent, and it is not thought to occur for genetic reasons.

Why should EDS or JHS contribute to the development of POTS? As I understand it, the theory goes something like this. EDS and JHS can cause POTS because the lack of adequate collagen leads in some way to 'lax' blood vessels and, by extension, compensative tachycardia. In other words, the general laxity of the skin in the person with EDS impacts, in turn, on the tautness of that person's blood vessels causing a degree of dysfunction therein. This in turn forces the heart to beat faster to compensate. If this is correct, then POTS would seem to be incurable for those who have EDS/JHS and POTS.

However, I seriously doubt the credibility of this theory. For a start, if it were true, then *everyone* with EDS would also have POTS. In other words, if a lack of collagen somehow produced the malfunctioning blood vessels we see in POTS, then for those with EDS *this should be true across the board*. Rather, only a small fraction of those with EDS also have POTS. Evidence from one study, by Jacob and Grubb, on the co-presence of POTS and EDS supports my view. They write:

"...The mean increase in heart rate after standing for at least 3 minutes was higher in (EDS) patients compared to controls (22 vs 15 bpm). Fifteen percent of hypermobile patients and none of the controls fulfilled the stringent criteria of postural tachycardia syndrome."[39]

In this study, therefore, only 15% of the EDS group had POTS. That number is simply too small to suggest that EDS somehow causes POTS - the percentage would need to be much higher before one could suggest that with any confidence. Furthermore, the mean increase in heart rate from supine to standing in the EDS group was only 22 beats, which is only slightly higher than the normal increase (10-20 BPM) in the healthy person, and the fact that it is slightly higher can probably be explained by the 15% of EDS patients in the study who did, in fact, have POTS (i.e. their presence in the study slightly 'skewed' the results). Furthermore, if there is something specific about EDS

---

[39] *ANS Primer*, chapter 111.

which contributes to POTS then why is it that there are so many people with POTS who *don't* have EDS? This last fact points to the root cause being something else entirely. Furthermore, if someone has EDS from birth and if EDS causes POTS, then that person should also have POTS from birth. But neither of these are true: only a tiny fraction of those with EDS have POTS and those who do have EDS from birth, do not also have POTS from birth - rather they develop POTS later. Indeed, I have not come across any case of POTS existing from birth.

It is my strong feeling that those who have both EDS and POTS have the latter for the same reason everyone else has it: due to a crisis in their brain after some kind of 'traumatic' event, broadly understood, including a 'humdinger' of a viral illness. If you are reading this and you have EDS as well as POTS, ask yourself whether there is more evidence for your POTS having been caused by a specific event which your brain might have perceived as 'traumatic' or whether you have had POTS for 'as long as you can remember', due to a genetic malfunction in collagen production. I suspect the former.

Other Limbic System Related Conditions Which Overlap with POTS Syndrome

In going through the various parts of the "POTS elephant" above, my aim was to suggest how each one of them can, in theory, be traced back to a limbic system in crisis. However, in addition to there being 'subsets' of POTS, it is also commonly noted that there are limbic system conditions with which POTS often 'overlaps'. I will now consider each of these in turn so as to illustrate how, in fact, these conditions too should probably not be thought of as 'wholly separate' conditions, but as stemming from the same root cause.

viii) *Irritable Bowel Syndrome (IBS)*

IBS need only be discussed briefly, as its causes, in light of limbic system malfunction, are obvious. They are the following: if the limbic system is in crisis, the autonomic nervous system is in crisis, and the sympathetic branch of the nervous system is favoured over the parasympathetic. It is the latter which is required for digestion. When the former is active, blood is drawn away from the internal organs, blood which is needed for efficient digestion and elimination. When this happens, all kinds of digestive problems emerge, as the body is simply not in a position to digest food effectively. Over time, coupled with increasing allergic responses (cf. the mast cell discussion above) the body becomes sensitive to various kinds of foods which previously would not have caused any problems. It is not uncommon for the POTS patient to have a highly restricted diet, and problems with nausea, vomiting, constipation and diarrhoea. All of these symptoms can be explained by the fact that the autonomic nervous system's efforts are engaged in primarily non-parasympathetic activities, and that, therefore, the body's 'rest and digest' function is compromised.

ix) *Multiple Chemical Sensitivity (MCS) / Environmental Illness (EI)*[40]

The limbic system is the part of the brain which, of course, processes smell. MCS, in its severest forms, is caused initially by an exposure to noxious chemicals. Following this initial poisoning, the limbic system 'rewires' itself (as part of a maladaptive neuroplastic response) to detect all chemicals as threatening. In addition, the sense of smell of the person with MCS becomes increasingly hypersensitive and they are able to detect smells that others cannot and at a level of intensity that others cannot. Exposure even to small levels of chemicals can lead to various physical reactions, including loss of voice, flu-like symptoms, migraines, nausea and, in extreme cases, anaphylaxis. We shall discuss MCS in more detail in the next chapter. For now, it is important to note that it is also possible to become sensitive to chemicals *without* having had an initial chemical poisoning. This is because the limbic system's various parts all inter-relate. The initial trauma - such as a virus - may be the cause for the limbic system crisis but, over time, that crisis becomes more and more severe as stress builds upon stress. The result is that the cingulate cortex, which processes smell in the limbic system, may eventually become adversely affected. At this point, chemicals might seem more overpowering than before and might lead to adverse reactions. Indeed, those with POTS often

---

[40] A specific and severe form of MCS which is well-known is 'Gulf War Syndrome' which affected soldiers in that conflict following chemical exposure.

report this increased sensitivity to smell (and also to sound and light), a further indication that there is a problem in the part of their brain which processes sensory experience, i.e. the limbic system.

x) *Chronic Fatigue Syndrome (CFS)/ Myalgic Encephalomyelitis (ME)*

Many patients with POTS are also diagnosed with CFS/ME or, alternatively, are diagnosed as only having CFS/ME and learn much later that they in fact have also had POTS all along. Indeed, there are cases to be found on the internet of those who have been disabled for years, decades sometimes, believing they have CFS, only to find they in fact have POTS as well. Furthermore, there are many symptoms which both conditions share and, indeed, one study suggests that up to 30% of those with CFS/ME actually have POTS. [41] The symptoms of CFS can include: overwhelming fatigue and exhaustion which cannot be explained by any other medical reason; memory impairment and problems concentrating; sore throat, muscle pain and joint pain (without swelling); severe headaches; sleep which is not restorative; post-exertional malaise; gastrointestinal disturbances; visual disturbances (blurring, light sensitivity, eye pain); chills and night sweats; orthostatic intolerance; dizziness, fainting and problems with balance; brain fog; allergies and

---

[41] As reported in the *Daily Mail*. See:
www.dailymail.co.uk/health/article-2659736/Third-ME-cases-wrongly-diagnosed-Experts-says-thousands-thought-chronic-fatigue-actually-similar-condition-treated.html

sensitivities to foods, odours, chemicals and medications, as well as anxiety, mood swings, irritability and panic attacks.[42] Given these symptoms - which no doubt will also be familiar to the person with POTS who is reading this book -, it is unsurprising that doctors unfamiliar with POTS would diagnose someone with these symptoms as having CFS. For all of these reasons, I believe it important to consider CFS in more detail.

Like POTS syndrome, the cause of CFS has not yet been established definitively (hence, once more, the word 'syndrome'), although, as with POTS syndrome, a virus often precedes it. As a result of this, it is often assumed - as in the case of POTS - that those with CFS are unfit following a period of bed rest after a viral illness, and need to pursue a reconditioning programme. I have argued that this deconditioning hypothesis is untrue as regards POTS patients. I wish now, albeit briefly, to do the same for CFS, as I believe that the limbic system in crisis is also the cause of this condition. This will be of interest to the POTS patient who has also been diagnosed with CFS, as you will see that targeting a change in the function of the root cause of both conditions - i.e. the brain - should arguably lead to the amelioration of both conditions.

An Oxford University study by Myhill et al., showed that there are high levels of 'mitochondrial' dysfunction

---

[42] This list is paraphrased from the work of Okamoto, Raj and Biaggioni in the *ANS Primer*, Chapter 110.

in patients with CFS.[43] Mitochondria are tiny organelles which power the transfer of *energy* throughout the human body. In the study, a patient's subjective sense of fatigue mapped onto the objectively measurable mitochondrial dysfunction in the patient. What this study did not really address, however, is *why* these mitochondria should begin to malfunction in the first place but rather seemed to assume that they had malfunctioned 'of their own accord'. But let us look at it this way: the proper functioning of mitochondria depends on the body's energy producing functions to be working properly. For this to happen, the autonomic nervous system must be in balance. If it is in a crisis state, then the body is stuck in chronic 'danger' mode, and both digestion and the absorption of nutrients are compromised. In such a state, the body *is not putting its efforts into creating energy*. If this is the case, then mitochondria simply cannot be produced properly and so the levels of mitochondria become low.

Limbic system crisis also explains why those with CFS are often sensitive to other viruses through a reduced immune system and also why, even when they do not have a virus, they often feel like they are perpetually 'coming down with the flu'. For, when the limbic system is in a crisis state, *it shuts down the immune system*, and this has a wide range of effects. Bruce Lipton explains why:

---

[43] For Myhill's paper, see:
www.ncbi.nlm.nih.gov/pmc/articles/PMC2680051/

"Why would the adrenal system shut down the immune system? Imagine that you are in your tent on the African savannah suffering from a bacterial infection and experiencing a bad case of diarrhoea. You hear the gutty growl of a lion outside your tent. The brain must make a decision about which is the greater threat. It will do your body no good to conquer the bacteria if you let a lion maul you. So your body halts the fight against the infection in favor of mobilizing energy for flight to survive your close encounter with a lion. Therefore, a secondary consequence of engaging the HPA axis is that it interferes with out ability to fight disease."[44]

If the brain is stuck in 'survival mode', then the immune system loses out in favour of the predominant sympathetic nervous system activity. A weakened immune system, as a result of overactive sympathetic activity in the limbic system, explains the 'flu-like' sore throat and muscles pains those with CFS so often have, and this, I believe, is why there is a widespread belief that CFS comes about because 'the virus is still within you'. Arguably, this is (usually, though not always) untrue: it only *feels* this way, because the immune system functions have been shut down and become dysfunctional leading to the perpetual presence of flu-like symptoms.

The other CFS symptoms can also be explained by a brain in crisis: memory and concentration problems are clearly neurological issues as are headaches;

---

[44] *The Biology of Belief* (2008), 119.

gastrointestinal disturbances are the result of an imbalanced nervous system (cf. the consideration of IBS above); sensitivity to light, smell and increased sensitivity to sound can be explained by the fact the limbic system processes perception and that a limbic system 'in crisis' will startle more easily; chills and night sweats by the fact that the limbic system controls temperature regulation; problems with balance by the fact that the limbic system has a role to play in motor function; anxiety, mood swings, irritability and panic attacks are all obviously connected with the limbic system. In fact, some studies have indeed connected malfunctioning of the autonomic nervous system with CFS. I quote Okamoto, Raj and Biaggioni: 'Newton et al. observed that 75% of patients with CFS exhibited symptoms suggesting autonomic dysfunction as measured by the Composite Autonomic Symptoms Scale (COMPASSS).'[45] In the UK, a doctor called Ashok Gupta, who himself had CFS, went on to put forward a limbic system hypothesis for its cause, as well as a recovery programme based on his insights, known as 'the Gupta Program'. There have, in fact, been several pioneering researchers who have put forward hypotheses in the past decades along these lines, including Jay Goldstein all the way back in 1996 (*Betrayal by the Brain: The Neurologic Basis of Chronic Fatigue Syndrome, Fibromyalgia Syndrome, and Related Neural Networks*) and others, but, for whatever reason, these lines of research, and treatments based on them, have not been developed further by researchers so as to become mainstream.

---

[45] *ANS Primer*, chapter 110.

I believe that, in the same way POTS should really be termed 'LSIND' (Limbic System Induced NET Deficiency), a more accurate description of CFS would be 'LSIMD' (Limbic System Induced Mitochondrial Deficiency). My aim in mentioning this is to reassure the reader who has POTS, and who has also been diagnosed with CFS, that addressing the root cause should form part of an effective treatment for both conditions. In fact, common sense dictates that it is almost certain that the POTS patient - regardless of whether or not they are diagnosed as having CFS - does also have poor mitochondrial function, given that an adequate supply of mitochondria depends on the nervous system being in a healthy enough state to produce them.

Fibromyalgia

Fibromyalgia, which literally means 'muscle pain', is another additional condition those with POTS are often diagnosed with. It involves many of the same features of Chronic Fatigue Syndrome, to greater or lesser severity, but the primary difference is that the person with Fibromyalgia is in *considerable pain*. The link with the limbic system is, once again, clear. You will recall that the cingulate cortex is responsible for processing pain (as in the example given earlier of the pain you feel when you stub your toe). When the limbic system enters a crisis state, its ability to process pain also becomes maladaptive: everything starts to feel painful - your feet on the floor, the chair you sit on, everything. Medical researchers have in fact established this for quite some time: what is termed 'Classic Fibromyalgia' is in fact a problem rooted in the brain's pain-processing centres.[46] Once more, therefore, if you are reading this and you have both POTS and Fibromyalgia, know that both arguably point to problems within the limbic system.

Overlapping Conditions: Conclusion

My aim in mentioning these four conditions which often overlap with POTS is to point out how they are actually just different branches of the same tree: they all stem from limbic system malfunction and, if the root cause is corrected, they can all potentially be treated effectively. Whereas my aim in the first part of this chapter was to explain the 'Whole Elephant' of POTS syndrome, my aim in this second part, was to show that there are not 'other elephants' in the picture either: CFS, Fibromyalgia, IBS and MCS can all be conceived of - broadly speaking - as parts of the same overall problem, even though they must necessarily differ in which parts of the limbic system are primarily impacted and in what way.

Why Have We Missed 'The Whole Elephant'?

I have now tried to explain the 'whole POTS elephant'. I have attempted to argue why limbic system malfunction, as a result of the varied ways it can impact the health of the body, can explain the different

---

[46] See: www.webmd.com/fibromyalgia/news/20131105/brain-scans-show-fibromyalgia-patients-process-pain-differently

'subsets' of POTS as well as similar, overlapping conditions. But why has the limbic system link not yet been the focus of research?

The modern medical method is unparalleled in the excellence of its research methodologies. Its great strengths include the ability to test and analyse specific parts of the body, and this is often critical. For example, there are millions of cancer survivors who owe their survival to the ability of a specific kind of drug to target a specific kind of cancer. However, at other times, this approach can lead to adopting too narrow a view of a condition so that its 'bigger picture' may become lost. This is, I believe, particularly true of POTS. The problem is this: it can be a mistake to think that the main reality of what is going on in a human body can be reduced to the actions of *one* specific part. The main reality of what is going on in a human body is in fact how a myriad of different parts *relate* to each other. The former is easily measurable. The latter is much harder to measure. In other words, research needs to be conducted in which *what is specifically going on with a certain body part can be understood as a scientific fact* but *also in which the scientific fact of how that part relates to other parts of the body is also considered*. To relate this to POTS in particular: yes, we know that NET deficiency is a factor but what other part of the body might be able to tell us *why*? Could there be a malfunction in another organ (i.e. the brain) that could explain NET protein deficiency as a 'knock-on' effect?

In POTS syndrome, there are many different 'parts' of the body which been identified as malfunctioning. However, the scientific research progresses on the assumption that, some day, *one* of these malfunctioning parts will indicate 'the' cause, and that there will be a drug to correct that particular part. Of course, this research has advanced our understandings of POTS hugely (for, without it, we would never have known of NET deficiency in the first place). But a 'bigger picture' approach is also needed in which the possible reasons for why *all* of these particular parts are malfunctioning is considered. It is only when this bigger picture is taken into account that one can see the role of the brain in the condition as a whole.

Key Points from Chapter Three

In this chapter, we have seen how the 'whole elephant' of POTS syndrome can potentially be explained through reference to a limbic system in crisis: NET deficiency, deconditioning, low renin and aldosterone (and resulting low blood volume), mast cell activation problems, and (perhaps) small fiber neuropathy in the extremities. In addition, I have discussed how both viral antibodies, as well as collagen formation problems (in EDS and JHS) should probably not be considered as causal even though they can co-exist with POTS. Then, I discussed how overlapping conditions (such as IBS, MCS, CFS and Fibromyalgia) can all also potentially be explained by reference to limbic system dysfunction. With this in place, we then considered why it is that the root cause of POTS syndrome has been missed, as the result of focussing too much on the pathologies of individual parts of the body, and not also on the relationship *between* those parts.

Chapter Four: Rewiring the Limbic System & A Biological Hypothesis for Recovery

If the hypothesis I have put forward is correct then, logically speaking, the following two things need to happen in order for the patient to recover from the most salient aspects of POTS syndrome:

i) the limbic system must cease to be engaged in a 'traumatic loop' and must return to normal, thereby leading to a normal 'signal' being sent to the nervous system via the HPA axis with the result that its functions too return to a healthy homeostasis

ii) the NET protein must heal and return to normal function, thereby leading to normal blood vessel constriction upon standing and resulting normalised heart rates.

In this chapter, I aim to explore how both of these can happen. As for the first, there is ever increasing evidence, in the form of testimonials and case studies (several of which are on the book's website, www.whatpotsreallyis.net) that the first of these can happen through the power of self-directed neuroplasticity, by which I mean specific exercises the patient can do herself to direct a change in brain function in the limbic system. In particular, I will discuss in this context, the development of the *The Dynamic Neural Retraining System* (DNRS), a six month intensive 'limbic system rewiring' programme, discussing the reasons for its development, its form and methodologies, its initial applications for Multiple Chemical Sensitivity, how these applications were also transferred to POTS syndrome, and why the program also potentially works for that condition. As for the second factor, the healing of the NET protein, I will present a 'biological common sense' argument that this will happen 'naturally' once the limbic system is restored to a non-crisis state. That is to say that the return of the nervous system to a healthy homeostasis will lead to the NET protein being 'replaced' - as it *has* to be - in the body's natural 'rest and digest' repair cycle. At the end of the chapter, I shall also consider how successful limbic system rehabilitation should also address other aspects of the 'whole POTS elephant' identified in the last chapter.

The Background to The Dynamic Neural Retraining System

The Dynamic Neural Retraining System is an intensive six-month brain rewiring program, taught through either DVD or workshop format. It was founded by Annie Hopper, a Canadian who previously worked as a counsellor. Its key hypothesis is that the limbic system can, through trauma (broadly understood to include trauma as a result of physical injury, illnesses, chemical poisoning/exposure, and traumatic psychological events), change drastically and begin to malfunction. In chapter two, I outlined the physical effects on the limbic system which 'trauma' can have, including radically altered sensory perception (particularly of sound, light and smell) and an overactive HPA axis via which stress hormones (particularly adrenalin) are released continuously. The six-month intervention targets the limbic system with specific exercises which are aimed at taking the limbic system out of this crisis state thereby restoring normal function.

The Story of Annie Hopper

The DNRS was not originally created with POTS syndrome in mind. Its founder, Annie Hopper, had suffered, rather, from Multiple Chemical Sensitivity (MCS).[47] Let us now consider her own story in more detail, and in particular the events in her life that led her to research a cure for her own condition. Doing so will further elucidate the nature of POTS syndrome.

Annie Hopper developed MCS over time initially as a result of her working environment in which there was poor ventilation, mould and a high level of VOCs (Volatile Organic Compounds) emanating from the furniture, carpets and paint. Over time, she found herself becoming sensitive to chemicals and perfumes. These would give her headaches. In addition, she started to have pains and aches throughout her body, which were later diagnosed as Fibromyalgia. After around a year of a slow but steady escalation in

---

[47] The following summary of Annie Hopper's story is adapted from the first chapter of her book, *Wired for Healing*.

symptoms, despite seeking the help of both standard medical care and alternative practitioners, as well as batteries of tests including a (negative) CAT scan for a possible brain tumour, her condition deteriorated sharply. Hopper describes the effect of MCS on her at that point as follows:

"I literally felt like I was being poisoned by everything around me. I could no longer wear my usual clothes because I was repulsed by the chemicals in the detergent residue, which had morphed into some kind of putrid and toxic smell. Chemicals in scented products...produced symptoms of headache, nausea, rapid heart rate, possible convulsions, difficulty breathing, cognitive impairment and loss of voice. This was followed by complete exhaustion, muscle pain and twitching, which could last for a number of days after any exposure."[48]

At this point, Hopper attempted to do what most with MCS are forced to do: *avoid all chemicals at all costs*. The result of this, however, was that it became impossible for Hopper to continue her work as a counsellor, as even the slightest scent on one of her clients' clothes would result in symptoms. Finally, Hopper's symptoms worsened further still, and she developed electro-magnetic wave sensitivity (EMF sensitivity), a condition similar to MCS, but in which the sufferer's limbic system has become so sensitive that it has started to 'pick up' electrical signals as well, and detect these as threatening. This forced Annie to

---

[48] 2014, 5.

leave her home and live on a houseboat for months, away from all chemicals and electricity. She was isolated, depressed and, in her own words, 'rapidly losing hope'.[49] These feelings of hopelessness were compounded by the fact that, as is the case with POTS syndrome, the prevailing wisdom is that there is no cure for MCS. Environmental doctors and patients alike view the condition as a 'toxic overload' syndrome, i.e. that there are too many chemicals and toxins 'inside you', and that the treatment for this is detoxification and avoidance. Hopper, however, did not believe this to be the root cause. As she puts it: 'The symptoms were so cognitive in nature that I just knew it has to be a neurological injury (brain injury) as opposed to a physical reaction like an allergy'.[50] This stands to reason. If a chemical is dangerous and overpowering to one person, *but not to another*, then it should be clear that, given that the chemical itself has not changed, that the brain of the former person has changed such that it perceives the chemical *in a different way* to that of the latter's. It makes absolute sense that the primary part of the brain that would be affected in this way would be the limbic system as it is the part of the brain concerned with ascertaining, as we have seen earlier in the book, how 'safe' smells are. If the limbic system becomes impaired, its ability to process smell will likewise become impaired.

---

[49] 2014, 9.
[50] 2014, 9.

Discovering Neuroplasticity: The Key to Changing the Brain

Hopper sensed that the brain must hold the key to her condition, but the task in front of her was no easy one. *How* could she get her brain's sensory perception, and threat mechanisms, back to normal? In order to find out, she researched the brain with great determination. She came across the emerging field of neuroplasticity, or how specific self-directed interventions can lead a patient to change his or her own brain in a targeted way. Hopper read of different applications of neuroplasticity, from 'rewiring' the brains of those with Obsessive Compulsive Disorder (OCD) [51] to stroke patients creating new movement pathways in the brain

---

[51] I include here, for those interested, more information about the neuroplasticity studies into rewiring the brains of those with OCD. Brain scans have shown that OCD develops as a result of the overactivation of the part of the brain known as the 'caudate nucleus', which is responsible for many functions, but one of which includes the simple ability shift one's attention one from thing to the next. In the person with OCD, it has been shown that the caudate nucleus gets 'stuck', unable to disengage from the worrying thoughts and compulsions. Dr. Jeffrey Schwartz of the University of Pittsburgh designed a mindfulness-based cognitive behavioural programme to treat OCD which entailed the patients gaining 'psychological distance' from their OCD, seeing it not as part of them but as the result of 'confused' overactivation of the caudate nucleus, and deliberately attempting to form new healthy behaviours whenever an OCD thought occurred so as to 'act back' on the brain and change its structure. And this is precisely what happened. After just eight weeks of practice, the activity of the caudate nucleus had quietened down. Their 'attention processing' part of the brain was acting closer and closer to normal. They had, therefore, successfully changed the *physical structure* of their brains, through discipline, commitment and knowing what to do.

so as to be able to bring 'dead' limbs back to life.[52] Having read of these kinds of cases, she felt that it *must* be possible to design an intervention for MCS. If stroke patients could learn to move their arm again, Hopper hoped that she could 'rewire' her brain so that its threat mechanisms - and particularly those associated with smell - could become deactivated and that her sense of smell might thereby perhaps return to normal. Although this *seemed*, from where she was, isolated and living on a run-down houseboat, an impossible task, Hopper knew that technically it was not. The brain is built to change: *it is a neuroplastic organ*. The reason Annie knew it was *possible,* even if it *seemed* impossible, to change her brain was because her research led her to the theory of "neurons that fire together, wire together". Let us now say a little more about this theory.

Each part of the brain is made up of "running programs" of neurons which have "fired and wired" together. The idea of neurons "firing and wiring"

---

[52] The use of neuroplasticity in recovering from the neurological effects of stroke also deserve further mention. For, in the case of recovering from stroke, it is not just a case of replacing one dominant set of neuronal pathways with another, for the affected movement patterns in the case of the stroke patient have actually been *destroyed*. The patient needs, therefore, to create new neurological movement patterns 'from the ground up'. Edward Taub of the University of Alabama at Birmingham designed an intensive rehabilitation programme called "C.I." or (*Constraint Induced Movement Therapy*). Patients, through repetitive exercises for up to eight hours a day initially, learn how to move the affected parts again, by 'acting back' on their own brains so as to change brain structure positively, creating new neuronal connections related to movement. Truly the brain is a neuroplastic organ.

together was first put forward by Donald Hebb, a Canadian neuro-psychologist, in 1949. We could also call these hardwired neurons 'brain circuitry'. These neuronal connections wire together as the brain develops and learns about the world and they concern *everything*: how we speak, how we move, how we think, feel and experience life. As the brain learns more and more about each of these domains (and many others besides), there forms dominant 'series' of neuronal pathways relating to each domain. These pathways determine how these functions take place. This is why each individual person will have *his* exact ways of moving, speaking, and experiencing the world, ways which will be subtly (or not so subtly) different from another's way of performing similar functions. For any given activity, then, the brain has developed countless 'dominant programs' of neuronal circuitry, each comprised of countless numbers of neurons which have 'fired and wired' together. What these "wired pathways" entail in practice is the fact that the brain likes to follow "the path of least resistance". It automatically goes to the brain programs and pathways which *are the most frequently exercised*.

Let's now apply these ideas to a limbic system in crisis. Hopper deduced that the most 'frequently exercised pathways' in her limbic system were those of threat and survival and that that was the case as a result of the initial chemical poisoning her brain had experienced. Furthermore, she deduced that if there were some way of 'exercising' the limbic system for long enough in non-threat and non-survival pathways, then it was conceivable that her limbic system might start to run on a new set of 'dominant', 'hardwired' and 'non-traumatic' pathways. In other words, by 'dampening' the heightened state of trauma in her limbic system, something which had led to the smell centres in her cingulate cortex becoming "supervigilant", she might, in turn, be able to reduce the hypervigilant sense of smell that a traumatised limbic system tends to have. In this way, Hopper was attempting to 'rewire' her traumatised limbic system using the *positive* principles of neuroplasticity (i.e. that there are specific targeted exercises we can do to change brain function) even though her brain had entered into such a crisis state thanks to the *negative* principles of neuroplasticity (i.e. in this case how the brain can change automatically and primitively as a result of a negative/traumatic experience). To return to the 'fired and wired' theory, we can put the same insights as follows. Whilst it may *seem* that our brains are 'stuck' in a certain way (i.e. certain brain programs/circuitry have fired and wired and are, therefore, 'dominant'), with enough perseverance and application it is actually possible to create new pathways that become hardwired and therefore 'dominant', with the old pathways, in fact, 'disconnecting' through disuse. The challenge therefore was to develop a program which could retrain the brain to recover from MCS specifically. She pooled all that could possibly help together, and set about following a self-devised program. Hopper found that following the method she devised at times felt like 'defying gravity'. Nevertheless, her health steadily improved over those six months, her sense of smell normalised, her limbic system calmed down, and, having completed six months of intensive brain rewiring, she no longer needed to do the practice anymore. Her MCS, EMF and Fibromyalgia were all gone and she had successfully 'rewired' her brain, returning her hypervigilant limbic system (and its smell centres) to normal function.

Methodologies of DNRS

Hopper identified the following twelve steps as being critical for rewiring the limbic system (I note here that these twelve steps are particularly pertinent to rewiring chemical sensitivity):[53]

1. Develop awareness of the expression of limbic system dysfunction in physical, psychological, emotional and behavioural patterns

2. Recognize and re-label symptoms as limbic system dysfunction

3. Interrupt patterns associated with limbic dysfunction

4. Decrease fear association to stimuli

5. Re-attribute symptoms to overactivated threat mechanism gone awry

6. Choose a new strategy for responding to stimuli

7. Cultivate a positive emotional state to dampen stress response

[53] 2014, 82.

8. Cultivate a positive psychological state to retrain thought patterns associated with catastrophic thinking
9. Incrementally train yourself to strengthen new brain pathways and to systematically desensitize your response to the triggering stimuli
10. Change habits associated with extreme harm avoidance and behaviour
11. Recognise improvements and celebrate them!
12. Repeat the new strategy daily for a minimum of an hour per day for 6 months "

The DNRS draws on many techniques to create exercises that speak 'in the language of the limbic system', utilising the limbic system's 'sensitivity' to events, experience, sensation and emotion in clever ways designed to 'lift' the limbic system out of a state of crisis. Whilst the DNRS exercises are 'psychological' in nature, these have been adapted specifically to 'speak' to a limbic system in crisis and, furthermore, the exercises are also performed with a level of repetition which is required to lift the limbic system out of that physical impairment. Indeed, the DNRS exercises are performed with a level of intensity that would not be seen in standard 'psychological' interventions.

The 'one hour a day' minimum point is also important for the reason just mentioned, namely that the aforementioned intensity of practice is required to 'lift' the brain out of a traumatic state. Whilst most who practice for one hour a day should recover, it is also notable that many participants spend two or three hours per day on the core practice, and a minority even practice for four hours a day, over six months. In the same way that it is hard work for a stroke patient to create new neural circuitry associated with movement, so too is it hard work to rewire the limbic system. Changes often, however, start to happen very quickly. Many with MCS report resolution of any major symptoms within a couple of months, weeks and, in some cases, days. Regardless of the speed of change, however, it is essential to maintain the exercises for six months so as to *hardwire* the changes in the brain. The discipline and commitment required are considerable, but the feeling of having put in the hours over six months, and the sense of having a 'new limbic system' after that time, is unparalleled.

The various techniques the DNRS has adapted to rehabilitate the limbic system include: cognitive behavioural therapy, neuro-linguistic programming, mindfulness based cognitive restructuring, emotional restructuring therapy, incremental exposure to context of perceived risk followed by brain retraining and behaviour modification therapy. As a whole, the program may be described, in Hopper's own words, as a '…top-down neuroplasticity-based psychoneuroimmunological intervention that assists in normalizing the threat and survival mechanism within the limbic system and downgrades the brain's maladapted chronic stress response.'[54] By "psychoneuroimmunological", Hopper means that it is a 'PNI' intervention:

[54] 2014, xi.

the health of the body (or its immunological state) changes in response to the change in the brain, or, more precisely, as a result of the calmer HPA axis signal being emitted to the rest of the body via the nervous system.

The Efficacy of the DNRS for Multiple Chemical Sensitivity

The DNRS was created relatively recently, with its DVD program only having been available since 2011 and, therefore, there has not been the amount of research into the program one might expect. This is now about to change, however.

A multi-stage academic research study by the University of Calgary, a leading university in brain imaging and brain research, and the University of Alberta, a leading university in researching integrative medicine, is seeking funding (as of early 2017) in order to test the efficacy of neural retraining for Multiple Chemical Sensitivity, Chronic Fatigue Syndrome and Fibromyalgia. This independent research study will include functional magnetic resonance imaging (FMRI) and various other markers in health at baseline and at six months post-treatment intervention in participants who are implementing the DNRS program. Researchers will assess scans and other markers to learn more about the potential impact of DNRS on the brain. The scans will identify what changes (if any) are occurring in the brains of DNRS participants and demonstrate how potential changes in brain function may relate to symptoms of illness. At the time of this book going to print, there has been the potential development that POTS may also be included in this study although this has not been confirmed. Readers are encouraged to visit the DNRS website for updates on this research.

Regarding other research, there was also an informal study[55] conducted by the DNRS itself into its efficacy which measured changes in multiple chemical intolerance (MCI) - a cluster of varied symptoms commonly found in MCS, CFS and FM. This preliminary data collection study made use of the 'QEESI' scale (Quick Environmental Exposure and Sensitivity Inventory), a standard scale used to assess severity of MCI developed by Dr. Claudia Miller of the University of Texas.[56] The QEESI scale operates on a scale from 0-100, where, for both symptom severity and chemical sensitivity, patients are graded as: 0-19 (low); 20-40 (medium); 40-100 (high). In order to be included in this study, participants had to have a score of 40 or over.

55 participants completed the QEESI scale at baseline and *at least at one point* in the next 3, 6, 12 or 36 months. The results were promising. On average, QEESI scores for "chemical sensitivity" decreased by 38 points, for "symptom severity" by 32 points, and for "impact on life" by 38 points. If one were to define "full

---

[55] This data was presented by Annie Hopper at the American Academy of Environmental Medicine Conference in October 2013. A YouTube video of that talk can be found here:
www.YouTube.com/watch?v=0_-nM2dHXMk (or look up 'Hopper AAEM presentation').

[56] For the scale, see:
www.institutferran.org/documentos/SQM/interpreting_QEESI.pdf

remission" from MCS as having a QEESI score of less than 20, then around 30% of the participants achieved full remission whilst another 20% achieved a "partial remission" QEESI score of less than 40. In short, slightly over half of participants achieved full or partial remission. 60% of participants improved by at least 20 QEESI points. However, four participants did not experience positive changes and two participants' symptoms increased in severity. In short, despite the limitations of this 'informal' study, there is strong initial evidence to show that brain retraining is an effective treatment for MCS. The study by the Universities of Calgary and Alberta, in any event, will give us more concrete data in the years to come.

I also note here that many case studies and testimonials have been gathered by the DNRS, often illustrating the before and after effects of taking the program. Those interested in watching videos of those who have recovered from MCS, and related conditions, using the DNRS should go to this link: https://retrainingthebrain.com/success-stories/. I will also be discussing three video testimonials of those who have used the DNRS to recover from POTS shortly.

What is the link between MCS and POTS?

Sometimes major breakthroughs in medical science happen 'by accident' and I believe that, one day, the fact that the DNRS is an effective treatment for POTS will be seen as one of those 'accidents'. For it was never originally intended for POTS, and yet it turned out to be effective for that condition also. This came about as several POTS patients who also had MCS took the DNRS program in the hope of curing MCS, but they actually ended up recovering from *both* conditions. It is notable, indeed, that many with POTS are also sensitive to chemicals and perfumes, as well as to sound and light, symptoms which indicate that the part of the brain responsible for processing stimuli, i.e. the limbic system, is in a crisis state. This points to the shared neurological origins common to both conditions and, had this 'accident' never happened, it is unlikely that others would subsequently have recovered from POTS using the program, thereby showing its potential efficacy in treating the condition.

There are, however, undoubtedly pertinent differences between the two conditions. One might hypothesise that the difference between the person who "primarily has POTS with MCS" and the person who "primarily has MCS with POTS" is a question of which parts of the limbic system are most affected. The severest symptoms of those patients whose cingulate cortex is most affected, i.e. the part of the brain associated with processing smell, are likely primarily to have chemical sensitivity with POTS as a possible secondary condition. Meanwhile, those patients whose hypothalamus is more affected are likely primarily to have POTS, as their HPA axis will be setting off adrenalin *all the time*, with MCS present to some degree. Obviously, in some cases, it is possible for both POTS and MCS to be present with the same severity and, in other cases, for someone to have POTS but not MCS and vice versa. My hypothesis, in short, suggests that both conditions involve limbic system dysfunction but which part of the limbic system is most affected will dictate whether the person primarily has POTS or primarily has MCS: the cingulate cortex is the part primarily responsible for MCS whilst the hypothalamus it the part primarily responsible for POTS.

There is, furthermore, another essential difference between the two conditions which needs to be kept in mind. And that is that although the root cause of POTS is in the brain, it also involves significant 'knock-on' changes in the body as a result of this neurological origin and, in particular, in the malfunction of the NET protein and resultant problems in blood vessel constriction. It is essential that patients recovering from POTS using the DNRS understand that they have a two-fold task in front of them. First, the brain needs to be rewired and, second, the NET protein needs enough time to heal. This is a noticeably different scenario from those with MCS for, although there are also widespread changes in the body as a result of MCS, these do not lead to NET deficiency and problems standing up. NET takes time to heal (how much time I will consider later in this chapter). Sometimes, there is confusion amongst POTS patients using the DNRS who are not experiencing the 'dramatic' reductions in heart-rate they hope for after a month or two of rewiring their brains and, as a result of this confusion, may quit the program even though they have started to feel much better. *It is essential to understand that the heart-rate will remain high (or relatively high) until NET has also healed.*

Three Case Studies of Those Who Have Recovered from POTS Using DNRS

Let us now consider three case studies of those who recovered from POTS using the DNRS (I use the first names only in two of these case studies so as to protect the privacy of those concerned).

Case Study One: Lauren Dinkel

Lauren Dinkel developed POTS after contracting mononucleosis at the age of 19. She had POTS for over four years before she found the DNRS. In the last of those four years, her condition had deteriorated to the point that she could not stand up at all, was in a 'tilt-in-space' wheelchair, in constant pain and unable to eat more than a handful of foods. Her heart rate in a *supine* position was around 135 BPM. Light and sound would give her migraines. Lauren's hair had begun to fall out, she had become skin and bones, and she had lost all hope. Her mitochondrial cell function was on the level of an elderly woman. Her family tried everything. Lauren visited over 35 specialists and countless alternative medical practitioners, and her parents spent over $100,000 outside of their medical insurance in trying to find the answer to their daughter's suffering. POTS was not the only condition Lauren was diagnosed with. She was also diagnosed with Fibromyalgia, Irritable Bowel Syndrome, Chronic Fatigue Syndrome, Multiple Sleep Disorders (including atypical narcolepsy), Pollen-Food Allergy Syndrome along with Mast Cell Activation Problems, Movement Disorder and Non-Epileptic

Seizures, Multiple Chemical Sensitivity, Electromagnetic Hypersensitivity Syndrome, Depression and Anxiety.

Lauren attended the DNRS workshop in April 2013. Within days, she was out of her wheelchair, and she *never* used it again. She applied herself with relentless diligence to the program and, although in the first few months, many things were still physically very challenging for her, the speed of her overall recovery was nothing less than extraordinary. Six months after taking the program, an orthostatic test showed that Lauren no longer had POTS, with a supine and standing heart rate *both* in the 70s. Lauren felt that she was "100% recovered" slightly under a year after taking the DNRS program. As of early 2016, Lauren no longer uses the DNRS program, is fully free from POTS, is happily married, and is the proud mother of a young, healthy boy. You can read more about Lauren and see her video testimonial on her own inspiring website, from which this brief case study draws: http://wheelchair torollerblades.com A video detailing her recovery can also be found on that website.

Case Study Two: Frances

Frances is a young Australian woman who had had POTS and MCS for 3 years and food allergies for 13 years. She developed POTS after contracting Lyme disease. Before taking the DNRS program, she was bedbound most of the time, could just about walk to the bathroom and back, and nearly all of her personal care was done by her parents. She compared this experience to being 'like a toddler again'. She was unable to tolerate any light or sound on her right side and she was also unable to eat a varied diet. Her chemical sensitivity also made it very difficult for her to see her friends as she would react to the scents on their clothing. As Frances puts it herself: "I was in so much grief for what I had lost".

Frances ordered the DNRS DVD program having heard about Lauren Dinkel's website, after which her sense of hope came back. As she started to practice the program, she also set small challenges, such as building up walking and practicing her brain retraining exercises around particular scents. After several months, she was walking 'heaps' and had taken up her ballroom dance classes again. After another period of several months, she felt she was 80% better but decided to attend the DNRS workshop program to help with the last stages of healing. For this, she flew, with her father, all the way from Australia to the US, something that would have been inconceivable before starting the DNRS program. Since then, she has improved yet further. She can now eat almost any food, including curries. Her smell sensitivity has 'hugely improved' and she can 'actually see how people enjoy' perfumes. Today, Frances is living a full life and is training to be a ballroom dance instructor. To see the video testimonial on which this brief case study is based, see: www.YouTube.com/watch?v=vJNuZY1u86Y&index=5&list=PLYJFpQmarJCCwEll3-6l0s2F3r8zCELEh (or look up on Youtube 'DNRS Frances POTS' - it should be the first search result).

Case Study Three: Brittney

Brittney was sick for four years. She was diagnosed with Lyme disease, POTS/dysautonomia, MCS, EMF, food allergies, PTSD, anxiety disorders and depression. She saw neurologists, cardiologists, endocrinologists, naturopaths and other alternative practitioners. She had a team of medical support and extended family support which meant that there was someone with her 24/7. At the worst of her illness, she did not see the outside of her house for over a year and a half. She spent over $300,000 in pursuing different treatments, some of which helped a bit but some of which also made her condition much worse. She was in tremendous pain, unable to stand, and she would go into convulsions if she attempted to walk. Interestingly, from the point of view of this book's hypothesis, she felt that her nervous system was 'constantly firing off'. She also had blurry vision and was unable to eat more than five particular foods for over 18 months. Her condition deteriorated to the point where any treatment or supplement might send Brittney to the emergency room.

Brittney ordered the DNRS DVDs having heard about Lauren's website. Within the first three to four days of practicing the program, her mood improved, and she no longer felt so 'stuck'. After several weeks, she was able to walk again, and she also gradually expanded her diet, gaining 15 pounds over six months. At that point, she attended the DNRS in-person workshop travelling *on her own*, reporting that her chemical sensitivity was 'completely gone'. She even had her first glass of wine in five years! She is now getting her life back, as she puts it, 'in ways I could never have imagined'. For the video on which this brief case study is based, see: www.YouTube.com/watch?v=57Y3_Ifq7VQ&list=PLYJF pQmarJCCwElI3-6l0s2F3r8zCELEh (or look up 'DNRS Brittney POTS' on Youtube - it should be the first search result).

These three testimonials have all been featured on the DNRS website and Youtube channel. Additional testimonials which I have gathered for the purpose of this book can be found on the book's website (www.whatpotsreallyis.net).

A Summary of the Biological Process of Recovery from POTS Syndrome Using the DNRS

I now present a hypothesis as to what changes occur in the person with POTS who takes the DNRS program.

As mentioned above, one must think of recovery from POTS as a two-fold process: the healing of the brain first and foremost and then the healing of the body (which can only occur as a result of the former) and, in particular, the healing of the NET protein. It is helpful at this point to remember that LSIND (Limbic System Induced NET Deficiency) is arguably a more accurate description than "POTS", as it captures the two key elements which need to heal: the limbic system first and foremost and then the NET protein.

The first important change which needs to take place, therefore, is that the hypothalamus in particular must cease to be in a crisis state and must cease to send alarm messages, in the form of adrenalin, down the HPA axis (hypothalamus-pituitary-adrenal gland axis), the most important pathology in POTS syndrome as identified in chapter two. Once this signal to release adrenalin all the time is stopped, then recovery is arguably assured: it is only a matter of time and practice to hardwire the changes into place over the remaining time left in the six months. Many will find that, with diligent practice at the beginning, the constant release of adrenalin will cease in a matter of days or weeks. Other changes which can happen quite quickly are reduced sensitivities to light, sound and smell, and improved digestion and energy.

Once the HPA axis has started to normalise, the second key stage of recovery can now begin as all of the normal functions of the autonomic nervous system will resume: energy production, digestion, the proper functioning of the immune, endocrine and thyroid systems, and more besides. As this healing takes place, *and it takes place slowly over months*, the NET protein should also begin to heal as part of the body's natural 'repair' cycle. Although it is not clear how long this will take, the NET protein *will* surely heal for, like nearly every other part of the body, it is constantly being replaced during the body's 'rest and repair' cycle. Furthermore, the NET protein is situated in 'soft muscle' which, of all muscle kinds, is the kind of muscle which the body renews and repairs most quickly. The NET proteins you had when you were five years old are not the same as the ones you had when you were seven, ten, fourteen or sixteen. It is constantly being renewed. The precise rate of NET protein healing needs to be determined by specialists but I suspect, from considering recovery stories from POTS using DNRS that it could take, at the least, three months and, at most, eight months. Neither are particularly long periods of time when it comes to recovering from an illness of such severity. Furthermore, there is reason to think that the patient can make a significant impact on the speed with which the NET proteins heal through diet. Indeed, it is not called a 'protein' for no reason! NET is made up of the same amino acids you eat in your beef, chicken or lentils. As long as the person recovering eats good food in copious quantities, NET should heal efficiently and relatively quickly. I will provide further considerations on the role of diet in the next chapter.

It is important to remember the fact that the process of NET healing will take several months. For this reason, although the patient should still feel *hugely* improved in the first months of brain rewiring, familiar symptoms may persist for several months albeit at lower levels of severity. In particular, the person recovering may still feel 'somewhat' shaky, curiously 'on edge' and, frankly, as if there happens to be extra adrenalin floating around their system, which there is as a result of NET deficiency. For some time, the heart will still beat somewhat faster than it should upon standing up. However, one's overall heart rates should become noticeably lower once the HPA axis normalises and the excess release of adrenalin ceases. By this I mean that, whereas before, someone might have had, say, a standing heart rate of 130 and a supine heart rate of 90, after the HPA axis normalises they should look forward to a standing heart rate regularly under 110, and often below 100, even if their supine heart rate is still 30 beats lower than that until NET heals. In addition, during the early stages of recovery symptoms may flare up every now and again, although these will not be as severe as before. It is imperative that these 'residual symptoms' are not misinterpreted as signs that the illness is returning: they are merely symptoms of the NET deficiency 'aftermath' of having had the limbic system stuck in a traumatic loop. It is also imperative that the patient continues rewiring her brain, as the brain must become as normal as possible, with any emotions, associations or memories concerning the traumatic loop becoming long forgotten. The job of the patient during this six-month period, therefore, is to keep their limbic system in good shape whilst the NET protein heals.

How does one know when the NET protein has healed fully? This will be known to have happened once the 'supine to standing' heart rate differential involves an increase of 10-20 beats consistently. (It is recommended that the person recovering take these heart rate measurements at the end of each month, but not more often than that, as continuous attention on the heart is not wise during recovery.) At that point, the NET protein will be working normally again, along with proper blood vessel constriction upon standing.

There are two other key things to point out at this stage. The first is that cardiovascular deconditioning will also be a factor in a higher supine-standing heart-rate differential. So it is conceivable that someone's NET protein may have healed up but their heart rate still increases from supine to standing by, say, 20-25 beats. It may be that this is just because of cardiovascular unfitness and it should reduce in time with sustained and sensible exercise. Such scores should be interpreted on a case-by-case basis. There will also, indeed, be a 'subjective' sense that NET has healed when the body feels less 'on edge'.

The second point is that although the NET protein is normally replaced in the body's rest and digest cycle, this cannot happen unless the limbic system crisis is stopped. This is because even though there is still some (albeit not particularly effective) 'rest and digest' functions ongoing in those with limbic system impairment, the NET protein cannot have a chance of healing until the waves of adrenalin reaching it are 'switched off'.

Why the DNRS is an Effective Treatment for the Other Parts of the 'POTS Elephant'

I consider now how the other symptoms and pathologies identified in chapter three should also potentially find an effective treatment in the form of the DNRS. Let us consider each other problem in turn:

i) *Deconditioning*. The DNRS, in and of itself, will not heal the person of deconditioning but will put them in the position of being able to engage in exercise again, which brain dysfunction and

NET deficiency currently render very difficult. Indeed, once the NET protein has healed up, the person should be in a position to start a proper exercise regimen again. This, in turn, will allow for cardiovascular reconditioning to boost heart size and blood volume.

ii) *Renin-Angiotensin-Aldosterone Problems.* Problems in the RAA network should resolve once the adrenal gland ceases to be overworked for, as we have seen, aldosterone is, in fact, secreted from the adrenal gland (in chapter three, I posited the idea that an overworked adrenal gland could no longer lead to sufficient aldosterone production). A healthy adrenal gland, in contrast, in time should produce normal amounts of aldosterone once more. This will have the knock on effect of allowing the body to hold onto sodium more easily (this being one of the functions of aldosterone) which will thereby address hypovolemia (low blood volume) naturally, given that salt is the primary substance that increases blood volume. The combination of this and cardiovascular reconditioning should lead to the complete return of normal blood volume. Furthermore, the fact that the RAA axis is itself 'intertwined' with the state of the limbic system, as we have seen in chapter three, should also indicate that a calm limbic system will lead to a calming of the RAA axis.

iii) *Mast Cell Activation Problems.* It is highly probable that problems with mast cell overactivation will also cease as, in the case of the POTS patient, the overactive limbic system has led to many 'false' - although physically very real - allergic (or "allergic-like") responses as a result of a chronic sympathetic state in the nervous system. As we have seen in the last chapter, one theory for MCAS problems in POTS patients, put forward by Prof. Raj, is the over-release of norepinephrine. It stands to reason that once this is over-release ceases and the whole system returns to homeostasis, then the incidence of Mast Cell problems should also be eliminated.

iv) *'Neuropathic' POTS Subtype.* My gut instinct is that the fact a sizeable minority of POTS patients have less sympathetic activation in the feet and lower limbs may be because those patients are the most deconditioned and therefore are those who are rarely upright (if at all). This has led to an element of denervation in the lower limbs due to a lack of circulation. However, it stands to reason that the nerves in the extremities of these POTS patients, once the root cause has been addressed and the patients become more mobile, will also heal, although this may take some time. I note though that this is conjecture on my part as I am unsure of the exact possible connection between limbic system impairment and small fiber neuropathy in the extremities.

v) *Irritable Bowel Syndrome.* Once the autonomic nervous system, which starts in the limbic system, has returned to normal function, the body will then be in a position to resume normal digestion with improved blood flow to the internal organs during parasympathetic nervous system activation or the 'rest and digest' phase of the autonomic nervous system, which is severely impaired whilst the limbic system is in crisis. For some with severe food sensitivities, however, this process will take months and involve, in some cases, the careful reintroduction of foods.

vi) *Chronic Fatigue Syndrome.* One of the central problems in CFS is mitochondrial dysfunction (mitochondria being the organelles which are responsible for energy supply)which is brought about by the inability of a nervous system 'stuck' in survival mode to produce adequate levels of mitochondria. It stands to reason that returning the nervous system to normal will allow for it produce energy normally once again and, therefore, for the number of mitochondria to increase.

vii) *Fibromyalgia.* The principal problem in fibromyalgia is over-activation of the limbic system's pain processing centres leading to widespread perception of pain throughout the body. Once the limbic system ceases to be in a crisis state, however, its pain centres' overactivation should also cease, leading to normal perception of pain.

In this way, not only should the HPA axis be treated effectively, but so too should the other 'subtypes' of POTS be treated effectively as well as other 'overlapping' limbic system conditions, either directly or indirectly as a result of brain rewiring.

Key Points of Chapter Four

The Dynamic Neural Retraining System, originally developed by Annie Hopper to treat another limbic system condition, Multiple Chemical Sensitivity, has also been shown - at an anecdotal level - to be effective for POTS syndrome. This indicates a similar neurological cause, although there are undoubtedly pertinent differences between MCS and POTS. The DNRS program utilises techniques which 'speak in the language' of the limbic system and which, with dedication and repetition, can lead the limbic system out of a crisis state, no matter what the initial cause of limbic system dysfunction was. The program works thanks to the science of neuroplasticity and the inherently malleable (changeable) nature of the human brain. Although the DNRS employs psychological techniques adapted for its limbic system rehabilitation purpose, the DNRS is not a 'psychological' intervention but an intervention to change the *physical* structure of the limbic system through focussed and intensive practice of techniques to 'trick' the limbic system out of its crisis state.

The DNRS addresses the root cause in POTS syndrome, i.e. limbic system dysfunction and, in doing so, leads to the normalisation of the autonomic nervous system, which itself starts in the limbic system. This, in turn, allows for the body's normal repair mechanisms to resume which, over time, should lead to the natural replacement of the deficient NET proteins, thereby leading to correct blood vessel constriction upon standing. Once this occurs the person is fully recovered from POTS/LSIND. The DNRS should also treat effectively other related conditions and/or so-called 'subsets' of POTS including problems in the Renin-Angiotensin-Aldosterone network (and resulting hypovolemia), Mast Cell Activation problems, Irritable Bowel Syndrome, Chronic Fatigue Syndrome and Fibromyalgia, in addition to paving the way for recovery from deconditioning.

Further Reading & Viewing:

Two excellent books, although not mentioned in this chapter, on the science of neuroplasticity in general are:

- Doidge, N., *The Brain That Changes Itself: Stories of Personal Triumph from the Frontiers of Brain Science*, Penguin, 2007.
- Doidge, N., *The Brain's Way of Healing: Remarkable Discoveries and Recoveries from the Frontiers of Neuroplasticity*, Penguin, 2016.

Annie Hopper's lecture, which presented the results of the informal data collection study into the efficacy of the DNRS for treating MCI (Multiple Chemical Intolerance), at the American Academy of Environmental Medicine Conference in October 2013 can be viewed here: www.YouTube.com/watch?v=0_-nM2dHXMk.

The DNRS website can be accessed here:
http:// retrainingthebrain.com

Chapter Five: A Potential Protocol For Recovery and Outline of a Trial to Test this Hypothesis

We are now in a position to put forward an outline of what kind of potential protocol could treat POTS effectively and what kind of research trial would be needed to confirm the ideas put forward in this book, if they are indeed along the right lines. Before doing that, however, I will first consider additional factors that might aid the recovery of the POTS patient, i.e. secondary measures that are probably also helpful to implement. These mainly consider the role of exercise and diet. That done, I then outline a potential protocol for the POTS patient to recover, which presents, in practical terms, the actions necessary to recover from limbic system crisis and to heal NET deficiency. Having put forward this protocol, I then suggest what data a clinical trial using such a protocol would need to capture in order to see if this protocol, and the hypothesis underlying it, are indeed correct. Of course, my suggested 'protocol' is just that, a suggestion, and as with everything else in this book, is not set in stone but could be refined and adapted as needs be.

The Role of Diet

Whereas brain retraining is essential for rewiring the root cause, diet is essential for determining the speed and quality of the return of normal NET protein function, the most important secondary factor in recovery.

Let us be clear, however, on two things. First, I note that for those with severe food sensitivities, it might not be possible to eat the amount or variation of food recommended immediately. Those for whom this is the case, should instead work on reintroducing foods one by one as their nervous system state normalises. Once their food sensitivities have considerably lessened, they can then consider incorporating the powerful principle which follows, namely of eating *food that is very good for you in huge quantities*. Even for those without major food sensitivities, it may take up to one or two months to build up your diet to the right amount of food and the right kind of food. Second, the NET protein will undoubtedly heal in any event as long as you eat a 'generally good' diet (it will probably heal up even if you just eat pizza and chips!). I say this so as to avoid the rise of any anxieties along the line of 'Will I recover if I don't follow the dietary recommendations?' Please remember that the following recommendations are aimed at *maximum healing efficiency* and that is all.

Now, onto those diet recommendations. Remember: the NET protein will be naturally replaced as part of your body's ongoing 'repair' cycle, once (but only once) your limbic system stress response is normalised (otherwise NET will remain 'swamped' by adrenalin and its repair will be impossible). How can we aid this process? The answer is by literally 'flooding' your body with the right nutrients, vitamins and proteins and in the right amount for maximum rebuilding at a cellular level. There is one diet in particular which I believe to be the best possible kind of diet for those recovering from illnesses where recovery requires this process of 'biological rebuilding'. It is called the *Wahls Protocol* diet.

The Wahls Protocol Diet

One of the most powerful examples of 'diet as medicine', the Wahls protocol was originally designed for multiple sclerosis patients. It was formulated by the medical researcher Terry Wahls M.D. who herself has that illness. (I note that, in discussing her diet protocol, I am summarising a freely-available TEDx talk Wahls gave in 2011, 'Minding Your Mitochondria'.[57]) Some of the worst physical symptoms of MS are caused by the reduction, by about a third, of a substance called 'myelin' in the brain - a protective layer that covers that organ. Despite receiving excellent conventional treatment, Wahls became more and more disabled in the five years following diagnosis and so she was determined to explore other ways of 'delaying the inevitable'. What she found in so doing however was something else entirely. Given her own background in medical science and research at University of Iowa Carver College of Medicine, she set about asking the

---

[57] Available here: www.YouTube.com/watch?v=KLjgBLwH3Wc

following questions: Of what is myelin composed? What foods could potentially, *if eaten in the right quantities*, rebuild myelin back to its normal size? Her answer was:

- 3 plates of fruit and vegetables every day
- a high quality source of protein at every meal and weekly organ meats
- a low carb, high fat diet along with no bread containing gluten

We might, similarly, ask: of what is NET composed? As mentioned previously, it is, of course, composed of protein. Accordingly, eating high quality protein in considerable amounts is recommended to aid your body in the repair process. The addition of the three plates of fruit/vegetables is also important however as, for various biological reasons, protein is best absorbed by the body when it is consumed in conjunction with the numerous vitamins and minerals which vegetables and fruit provide. I note at this point that a very helpful resource for the healing power of food is Murray and Pizzorno's *Encyclopedia of Healing Foods*.

The key point about Wahl's diet, in addition to the fact that she only ate food that is obviously good for you, are the *quantities* involved: three heaped plates of vegetables and fruit every day, for example, is no small task. But this was the definitive factor in leading Wahls to recovery. Indeed, she had already been eating a healthy diet in the five years previously. The only difference now was that she upped the *amount* she was eating, so that she was giving her body enough 'raw matter' to really rebuild. *She stuffed herself with the good stuff so that her body could literally rebuild itself.* Note, furthermore, that the diet does not necessarily involve supplements. Wahls found that, whilst supplements slowed her decline, it was only when she switched to getting the right amount of nutrients her body needed to rebuild her myelin levels from her food alone, that she got better. Your body wants the real McCoy, not pills.

The result? After just three months on this diet, Dr. Wahls could suddenly walk again after five years in a wheelchair. It was as simple as that: one day, she got out of her chair and could walk with the help of her cane. Within six months, she no longer needed her cane and after two years, she went horse riding in the Canadian Rockies. Her myelin levels had returned to normal. *She had physically rebuilt the myelin around her brain.* She still has MS, but she can live a normal life again: walking, swimming, running and going wherever she likes. She bikes the five miles to work every day. She subsequently developed the Wahls protocol diet and is developing trials based on her methods, including one, on the effect of the Wahls protocol on fatigue in MS patients, with good results.[58]

The actual scientific reasons for how Wahls, and others with MS, have been able to rebuild the myelin around their brains concern a kind of cell called the 'mitochondrion', a cell which we met earlier in relation to Chronic Fatigue Syndrome. Countless mitochondria

---

[58] See: http://terrywahls.com/research-update-full-edition/

are in your body, and their job is to transport energy around for all kinds of biological processes. If you eat the kind of diet Wahls recommends, these mitochondria become 'supercharged' to carry out their work. Once this happens, everything in your body rebuilds at a quicker biological rate than normal, and with far better *quality*. The body is remodelled on a cellular level. For our purposes, the more you feed your mitochondria, the more efficiently NET protein function will rebuild and, also, with much greater quality. However, unlike the MS patient, who must follow the Wahls protocol forever to maintain its results, the POTS patient, once NET function has returned to normal can afford to eat a 'generally' healthy diet, not worrying too much about quantities. *Once NET has normalised, it has normalised*. You may, of course, wish to keep up such a diet regardless: its health benefits will reach far beyond the NET protein, and will ensure excellent biological change on many levels. Most of your body, in fact, is replaced over a seven-year period. The quality of that change depends largely on what you eat. By eating well, and changing your limbic system, you will be - in a way - 'resetting your body': no small feat!

In my own recovery, I did not follow the Wahls protocol to the letter but rather took its general principle of eating more than I usually would. For around eight months, I:

- ate a high-quality source of protein with all three meals

- had two-three heaped plates of fruit and vegetables every day at a ratio of around 1:2 (I sometimes had a smoothie in addition as it was not always possible to reach the three-plate target through the main meals alone)
- tried to have organ meats at least once a week (liver, kidneys)
- did not have sugar, cakes, desserts save on very special occasions. I avoided alcohol completely.
- I had home-made bread, rather than cutting out on bread completely

By following these principles - or similar principles - for a sustained period of time, the POTS patient will efficiently and effectively be giving their body the tools it needs to rebuild NET function (and many other functions besides), allowing for a speedier recovery. Those interested in finding out more about the Wahls protocol diet should see the references at the end of this chapter. I note here that in making this recommendation I do not benefit in any way. I merely made use of the Wahls protocol myself as it seemed well-suited to aid me in the task of rebuilding my body. The general principle, however, *is to eat copious amounts of food that is good for you*.

In sum, by normalising the limbic system through the DNRS system, the NET protein should be replaced as part of the body's *rest and repair* cycle. This can only happen once the sympathetic and parasympathetic branches of the nervous system are in balance. Once the limbic system is rebalanced, NET healing is arguably guaranteed but the person recovering can aid its healing through eating an excellent diet in large quantities over a sustained period long enough to effect that required biological change.

Essential Additional Points About Diet: You Must Avoid Caffeine and Sugar

Both caffeine and sugar are absolutely out of bounds during recovery. There is a simple reason for this.

To consider caffeine first. Caffeine leads to the automatic release of adrenalin. That's right: if you drink caffeine, it forces your body to release adrenalin, and you have no say in the matter. Drinking caffeine is like drinking POTS! It also constricts blood vessels, including those to your brain, leading to a marked reduction in blood flow to the brain. This does not make your brain rewiring exercises any easier as it helps to be as clear-headed as possible during them.

Similarly, sugar (the kind found in processed foods - chocolate, cakes, sweets etc) also (although in a rather more round about way) leads to the release of extra adrenalin. This kind of 'empty calorie' sugar causes insulin levels to fall. The body aims to rebalance this state of affairs *by increasing adrenalin levels* so as to draw out glucose from the liver. So: eating sugar is also the same thing as eating POTS!

Put in this way, I hope that this is enough of a deterrent for you to avoid both caffeine and sugar during your period of recovery. Before starting the DNRS, indeed, it might be wise to reduce and eliminate your sugar and caffeine consumption over a period of a month or so (or go cold turkey on both, depending on what works). It does not help to have additional adrenalin floating around an already over-taxed system if it can be avoided.

The Role of Exercise

Whilst, according to the hypothesis put forward in this book, deconditioning is not the root cause of POTS, we do know that deconditioning plays a large role in the POTS patient's condition. Cardiovascular reconditioning will, therefore, be an important part of recovery, and this will almost certainly apply to every POTS patient, even if they have only had the condition for a short period of time. Basically, cardiovascular reconditioning is an important 'secondary' aspect of recovery.

The main question is when such a cardiovascular reconditioning programme should be commenced or, to put it another way: there is no point running before you can walk. Indeed, common sense would dictate that it would be wise not to commence any intensive cardiovascular programme until the NET protein has healed as, until it does heal, the heart has enough to deal with as a result of the blood vessel constriction problems. However, the person recovering should still build up sensible, moderate exercise in the early months of healing, as able. For example, if the patient has been very deconditioned, then a daily five minute walk in the first week, a ten minute walk in the second, fifteen in the third and so on, might be a good idea.

Other light activities such as gardening are also recommended for this time. Overall, a sensible aim during the first six months of brain rewiring would be to reach the point where it is possible to do an hour's daily walk without difficulty in addition to work around the house/garden and going shopping, etc. The increased circulation which these walks will bring will also aid in the recovery process. When the person recovering from POTS begins her walks, it is important not to worry about any minor 'on edge' symptoms: these are just the result of NET not quite having fully healed and the resulting spill over of adrenalin. Indeed, the exercise you are doing (as long as it is not overly intensive) is only helping along the recovery process of NET. This goes only for 'minor' symptoms though: listen to your body and if you need to rest, rest. It is also common if someone does an amount of exercise that is 'too much', especially at the beginning, that their heart rate will be elevated. If you notice your heart "thumping away" after exercise that day, know that this is not a sign of POTS returning but rather it is probably a sign that you should reduce the intensity of the exercise you are currently taking. It is helpful in such circumstances to remember the maxim: *'Just because you cannot do it today does not mean you cannot do it someday'*.

In addition, after several months of brain rewiring and when the time is right, the person recovering could also start to introduce all-round body strength training, as is right for the individual, given age and other circumstances. Whether this involves lifting weights in the gym, yoga, pilates, or body-weight exercises, should be a decision reached between the person recovering, her consultant and a physical therapist who specialises in reconditioning after illness. The same point applies: start slowly and build up.

As regards more intensive cardiovascular reconditioning and strength training, the one rule I would suggest is that the NET protein should have shown signs of being healed. The person will know this to have happened based on two things. First, there will be the subjective feeling that the sensations of 'being on edge' have gone. Secondly, there will be the objective measurements of the supine to standing differential. If this has returned to the normal 10-20 beats consistently, then NET has healed. Having said that, it is possible that NET may have healed fully even if the supine-standing differential remains in the 20+ beats per minute range. This is because deconditioning also plays a role in this differential and it is possible for NET to have healed but for the patient to be cardiovascularly unfit, such that their heart still increases more than 20 beats per minute upon standing (but less than 30). Prudence and sound judgement of each patient on a case-by-case basis should be employed.

A Short Note on Breathing

The following note is more conjectural but potentially important in the light of the impact of autonomic nervous system dysfunction on breathing. When our systems have become stressed, we tend to "over-breathe" and even to hyperventilate. If you suspect this to be the case for you, then it may be important to investigate ways to correct this, and to relearn correct breathing: nasal-only, soft, quiet, gentle and diaphragmatic (as can be observed in babies). Soft and gentle breathing, paradoxical though it may seem, leads to far grater oxygenation of the body than taking audible and big breaths, especially those through the mouth. The Buteyko breathing method may be helpful in this regard. I am only beginning to look into this myself, but Patrick McKeown has several helpful books on the method which may be of interest and which may act as another supportive secondary aspect of recovery.

The Role of Medicine and Drugs in Recovery

It is here especially that those medical researchers working on POTS syndrome could design a sensible plan for making use of drugs to reduce symptoms whilst also designing a sensible plan to withdraw those drugs when the time is right. I am not in a position to comment much on this but it would seem to me there could be a role for beta blockers in the first few months of brain rewiring to 'take the edge' off the extra adrenalin floating around and also to give the heart a slightly easier time. In addition, it would seem that the use of Flurinef - a synthetic replacement for aldosterone - should be monitored especially as, once the limbic system normalises, the body should start to produce aldosterone in the right amounts again (and, indeed, the whole renin-angiotensin-aldosterone network should normalise). I say that this should be monitored as the body's own normalisation of the RAA axis would, in addition to taking Flurinef, potentially lead to too much aldosterone in the system. Since aldosterone is one of the body's primary substances which retains salt, too much aldosterone could lead to too much salt retention and, by extension, high blood pressure. Similarly, once the RAA axis begins to normalise and the body begins to be able to hold onto salt naturally again, then taking extra salt ('salt-loading') may also be unwise and lead to too much salt in the blood. Therefore, it seems that a sensible withdrawal/tapering program should be devised for salt loading and Flurinef usage.

Bringing it All Together: A Potential Template for a Patient Protocol

These extra 'secondary' considerations in place, we now come to the crux of this chapter: a potential template for a protocol to treat POTS, which is divided into two six month phases, the first being rewiring the brain and the second being cardiovascular reconditioning. It may be that certain patients may need to spend more time on phase one, especially if they have other limbic system related conditions which are also severe. On the other hand, even those with the most severe limbic system conditions can recover in the six month period, and so it seems that the previous severity of the condition is not necessarily a good benchmark for determining the speed at which recovery takes place.

Phase One: Rewiring the Brain

- *Months 1-6*: Brain rewiring for at least one hour per day with graded exercise (cardiovascular and strength training) as able and cutting out all foods which will not aid recovery. Once food sensitivities are no longer an issue, aim for three plates of fruits and vegetables per day and a high quality source of protein with every meal and continue this for six months.

The key aims of this period are two. The overall aim is to *have the limbic system operating in a new non-crisis mode and to keep it there*. 'Keeping it there' is important, as this change needs to become permanent. The person recovering should not stop once they start to feel much better but continue their rewiring for the full six month period or as long as is necessary.

But the most paramount aim of all concerns the first month and that is to 'switch off' the over-supply of adrenalin and the feeling that the nervous system is constantly 'firing off'. For *once the adrenalin over-supply is turned off, the recovery process is on firm ground.* For this reason, I recommend the patient consider two hours of brain rewiring per day for the first two months or so. The reason for this is that this adrenalin 'switch off' can, in fact, happen really quickly, even within a matter of days or weeks. Once this happens, it is important to solidify this change. Two hours is just a recommendation however, and one hour a day should still guarantee recovery. In any event, once the adrenalin supply ceases, the NET protein will no longer be being overwhelmed by adrenalin and will be in a position to start being repaired naturally by the body. The person recovering will feel so much better once this 'oversupply' of adrenalin ceases. Their blood stream will have less adrenalin in it, they will feel less on edge, and they will have more energy. They will still feel somewhat 'shaky', as the NET protein is still deficient, but the actual continuous supply of norepinephrine will have ceased, leading to much less adrenalin 'floating around' overall.

Phase Two: Becoming Strong

- *Months 7-12*: Assuming normalisation of limbic system and evidence of NET healing, brain rewiring now becomes optional, but many may wish to continue albeit at a slower rate (say 15-30 minutes a day). The primary focus now is on a thorough - yet sensible - cardiovascular exercise programme designed by an expert, along with more advanced muscle strengthening. Once a full six months of the 'copious good food' diet has passed, the recovered person can instead switch to eating a 'generally good' diet.

The aim of this period is to regain full cardiovascular conditioning, thereby treating the secondary aspects of deconditioning, and to bring about continued positive biological changes in the body through diet. The DNRS can be employed as needed/as desired by the individual. Many find that, regardless of recovering from limbic system conditions, the program is helpful for everyday life.

What Would a Research Study Need to Show in Order to Prove the Hypothesis Put Forward in this Book?

A research study which expanded upon the hypothesis put forward in this book, refined it, tested it, and created a definite treatment plan based on it, would undoubtedly be a considerable undertaking, both in terms of financial resources and time. The potential rewards, however, are significant for the millions of those worldwide who suffer with POTS. Furthermore, although it would be a significant undertaking, the actual measurements needed to be taken during such a study in order to prove or disprove this hypothesis would be fairly straightforward.

In particular, the following tests would need to be made, both at baseline and six months later:

1. A tilt-table test
2. NET protein function test
3. Levels of norepinephrine/adrenalin in the blood stream in both supine and standing positions
4. Renin-Angiotensin-Aldosterone Function Test
5. Levels of Electrolytes, including sodium
6. Tests for Mast Cell activation problems
7. Quality of Life Questionnaire

A potential study would require a sizeable number of patients so as to get a sense of the DNRS success rate for POTS. Ideally, the various 'subtypes' within POTS should all be represented so as to ascertain whether or not limbic system impairment may nevertheless be the root cause no matter what 'subtype' one might have. The study would require those in the field of limbic system dysfunction rehabilitation at the DNRS, led by Annie Hopper, to work with expert consultants in the field of dysautonomia. The start of the six month trial could involve an intensive, POTS oriented workshop, led by Hopper and POTS consultants working together, teaching the DNRS methods, as well as other experts teaching the importance of diet and graded exercise. The following six months would also need to make use of an online support forum for those in the study, both to support each other and to ask questions of DNRS coaches as well as POTS consultants. Regular Skype calls for each patient with a DNRS coach, with a specialist in graded exercise and with a POTS consultant would also be important. Finally, those recovering should keep a log of the number of hours spent rewiring their brains daily, exercise taken and foods consumed, so that the results of their specific efforts could be mapped onto the objective results at the end of the six month period.

If, at the six month mark, the tilt table test, NET protein function, levels of norepinephrine in the blood stream, aldosterone and sodium levels are all normal, and if there is an absence of mast cell problems, then it will be clear that limbic system impairment is the cause of POTS and that limbic system rehabilitation is a very effective form of treatment. If not, then the search continues!

Conclusion: Over to You, Researchers!

My part in attempting to unravel POTS syndrome has now come to an end. I have presented what I believe to be the only logical explanation for the condition. I believe that limbic system dysfunction can explain most of the consistent findings medical researchers have found to exist in POTS patients and in particular the most important one of all for blood vessel dysfunction in POTS, namely NET deficiency. But it can also potentially explain low blood volume as a result of low aldosterone levels as well as mast cell activation problems, in addition to explaining why POTS patients are often unable to engage in exercise without great difficulty. Furthermore, the fact that a sizeable number have recovered from POTS by rewiring their brains, including from *very* severe POTS, indicates that brain retraining must hold the answer to treating the condition effectively. The testimonials on the book's website (www.whatpotsreallyis.net) provide additional anecdotal evidence for this claim.

The biggest obstacle to the hypothesis that I am putting forward may be the understandable fear that it is suggesting the cause is psychosomatic. At numerous points in the book, I have tried to counter this idea strongly, but I'll repeat the argument one last time: The limbic system is primitive, reacts in automatic ways and is very vulnerable to various kinds of trauma and it is never the fault of the individual concerned when they suffer a limbic system impairment. Indeed, how *could* it be their fault if a severe viral illness leads to the limbic system impairment? It is essential to remember that the constant release of adrenalin that the POTS patient feels is not a sign that they suffer from a psychological problem, but rather that they are suffering from the after-effects of a 'traumatic assault' (broadly understood) on their limbic system of an immense magnitude. The limbic system may be implicated in both anxiety disorders and POTS syndrome but *this is not the case for the same reasons*. There is more than one way for a limbic system to enter a crisis state and this point cannot be forgotten. Of course, it is possible for psychological conditions to co-exist with POTS, just as they can with any illness, and psychological problems - including depression and anxiety - may understandably develop as a result of having such a debilitating condition. But these should be seen for what they are: secondary problems.

Another obstacle may be the idea of using a 'mind-body' program to treat the condition. Researchers may worry that they are trying to cure people via a 'placebo' effect. Whilst understandable, I believe that this is also a misguided concern. This is not the same kind of scenario as when someone attempts to use a mind-body program to heal from an illness rooted only in the body itself. Rather, this is a case of people using a mind-body program to treat *the mind itself, the brain itself*, a very delicate organ that had been pushed into a state of crisis following a devastating event, through no fault of its own and through no fault of the individual concerned. This is not a 'placebo' scenario: instead, it is a targeted intervention aimed at a part of the brain itself that is crying out for help.

In addition, researchers may also find the DNRS exercises to be too simple and may dismiss them out of hand for this reason. To this I respond: they are simple for a reason. The limbic system cares about simple things, and so to lift it out of a state of trauma it needs to be treated on *its* terms. The limbic system does not care about the nuances of complex theories about NET protein deficiency or low aldosterone levels: indeed, it does not give a 'flying monkeys' about any such things! *All it wants to know is that life is safe again.* The DNRS exercises achieve this in very clever ways that have been very much adapted to what an impaired limbic system needs.

Finally, if there is still hesitancy amongst medical researchers regarding testing the efficacy of a mind-body program as a treatment for POTS, I would simply ask this: if it is true that the root cause of the condition is limbic system impairment (and it risks too much to dismiss this idea), then what other possible way *would* there be to treat it?

Although I am happy to raise awareness of the possibility that POTS is caused by limbic system impairment, I am not in a position - nor do I have the pre-requisite skills - to do more than that. The only people placed to test this particular hypothesis are specialist researchers and those at DNRS. If there is a researcher out there who reads this book and who wishes to expand on this hypothesis further, refine it and test it, in conjunction with Annie Hopper at the DNRS, then I invite them to do so, provided acknowledgement of this book is given. Also, I would be very happy to discuss the ideas put forward in this book with any medical researcher potentially interested in exploring them, if that might be helpful.

And if someone is reading this who themselves has POTS syndrome, whether or not a research study has yet taken place, you may wish to consider whether the hypothesis put forward in this book convinces you and, if so, take the step of purchasing the DNRS DVDs. If brain retraining does work for you - as I sincerely hope it will - then your story too will add to the mounting evidence that POTS syndrome may not need to be a 'syndrome' anymore.

One day, I hope it will be classified for what it is, namely a neurological problem, probably better described as *Limbic System Induced NET Deficiency*, along with the advice given to all those who suffer from it that there is a concrete and effective form of treatment.

Key Points of Chapter Five

In this chapter, I put forward a potential template for recovery from POTS, a template which is divided into two phases - rewiring the brain for six months, alongside a healing diet and building up basic cardiovascular fitness, and a second phase with optional brain retraining, alongside a healing diet and more intensive cardiovascular reconditioning. The role of diet and exercise as important secondary factors in recovery were also considered and the various suggested tests which specialists would need to undertake to test the hypothesis put forward in this book were presented.

Further Reading & Viewing

For more on the Wahls Protocol Diet, see:

> - 'Minding Your Mitochondria', TEDx talk on YouTube:
> www.YouTube.com/watch?v=KLjgBLwH3Wc
>
> - Wahls, T., *The Wahls Protocol: A Radical New Way to Treat All Chronic Conditions Using Paleo Principles*, Avery, 2014.

For the power of food to heal the body:

Murray, M., Pizzorno, J., *The Encyclopedia of Healing Foods*, Atria Books, 2005.

On the science of exercise:

Reynolds, G., *The First 20 Minutes: Surprising Science Reveals How We Can Exercise Better, Train Smarter, Live Longer*, Plume, 2013.

Addendum: General Points About Recovery and the DNRS Program

Scepticism: There are few who start the DNRS program who are not highly sceptical that it will work. This is largely because those with limbic system conditions have exhausted many other treatment options, have often been unwell for a long time, and are therefore understandably hesitant about believing that recovery is possible. The scepticism may be compounded by the fact that the DNRS exercises might seem 'too simple'. In response to the former, the point to bear in mind is that the brain is a highly neuroplastic organ and, if it is targeted in the right way, those new changes can 'come online' really quickly. Nearly all who recover using the DNRS would describe the changes it brings as being 'miraculous'. But they are not in fact miraculous, but rather an indication of how highly changeable our brains are (with a little dedication, that is). Indeed, the brain often changes quickly enough to enter into a state of limbic system impairment following a trauma. That is a maladaptive neuroplastic response. But with the right tools a healthy neuroplastic response can likewise be elicited surprisingly quickly. In response to the second point, the DNRS exercises are indeed simple (although not simplistic), but they are also aimed at a part of the brain which has a simple and primitive view of the world. Any exercise which attempts to 'rewire the limbic system' needs accordingly to speak in its 'language'.

My POTS came about as a result of an illness: is a 'psychological' treatment really going to help? In response to such an objection, there are several points to be made. The first is that the DNRS may employ techniques otherwise used in psychological settings, but it does so in a way that specifically speaks to the limbic system and at a level of intensity which is able to effect a limbic system change. Each time the practice is employed, millions of the 'right neurons' fire in the limbic system, changing its structure. In the same way that a stroke patient doing targeted exercises can rewire his brain to recover movement, so too can someone with the right exercises target limbic system function. Secondly, the brain may have entered a crisis state as a result of the body-mind connection, i.e. distress signals the brain received during the illness which 'tipped' it into an impairment, but it is the mind-body connection which can, with dedicated practice, lift that individual's limbic system out of a traumatic state. You did not contract POTS from thinking the 'wrong kinds of thoughts' - that would be ludicrous - but the right kind of thought with enough repetition and intensity can heal the limbic system.

Indeed, it should be emphasised that the DNRS *never* suggests that a patient has developed their condition through 'thinking negative thoughts', or other similar ridiculous claims. The limbic system conditions discussed in this book are never psychological in origin, but very physical conditions. As Hopper writes:

"Limbic System Dysfunction is located in the brain but the related conditions are far from being 'psychological' issues. They are trauma-induced brain impairments that affect many systems of the body. These conditions are physical in nature, they are real, they are painful, they are life altering, and they can be life threatening. Let me repeat: You are not alone, you are not crazy, and it's not your fault."[59]

In other words, the claim is that the brain of the person with limbic system impairment has entered a traumatic state *through no fault of their own.* The DNRS, however, offers tools which speak in the language of the limbic system to lift it out of a crisis state no matter how it entered into that state in the first place. No matter what the cause, the DNRS practices are aimed at 'tricking' the patient's limbic system out of a crisis state.

The Recovery Process: It is important not to read signs of relapse into any minor symptoms during the recovery process. Rather, recovery will initially proceed on a 'two steps forward, one step back / one step forward, two steps back' basis. This is natural to recovering from any condition and POTS is no different. The person recovering should be kind to herself during any setbacks, commit to the brain retraining, and understand these to be normal parts of the process. It is also helpful to understand that NET

---

[59] 2014, xx.

deficiency will continue for several months, thereby resulting in a slightly unusual 'on edge' feeling. You may feel 'odd' or 'peculiar' at these times. These sensations will reduce over time. Similarly, on rare occasions, minor chemical sensitivity or sensitivity to other stimuli may return. These incidents should also reduce with time and practice. Finally, mitochondrial dysfunction will also continue for several months, and so the person should pace herself carefully, so as to avoid 'crashing'. There will come a point where the 'ebb and flow' of recovery essentially ceases, and there is only an uphill curve.

Knowing that it is Impossible to Stick to the 'Ideal' All the Time: The above template for recovery is the 'ideal' template. No one will be able to stick to it all of the time, as human beings are not automated 'bots'. We all fall down and have to pick ourselves back up again. The thing to remember is that if you aim at the ideal but only manage to stick to the above template around 70% of the time overall, you should still make a flourishing recovery. Having said that, do cultivate an attitude of discipline. It may be helpful to have specific times established in advance when you will drop whatever else you are doing and perform the DNRS exercises. In my recovery, I kept a quasi-monastic schedule: an hour at 8 AM, 45 minutes at midday, 45 minutes at 5 PM and 20 minutes before bed. It really helped me to establish this routine.

Use of Technology During Recovery: Having a clear mind is important during recovery, as the exercises require considerable cognitive involvement. The constant use of screens and pinging of emails are not conducive to this. I found my DNRS practice was much improved on those days when I limited myself to one period of an hour online per day, and was even better on those days when I did not use the internet at all. This is a highly subjective piece of advice but others might find it helpful to follow. Limiting technology during recovery time is also helpful as it instils a sense of simplicity, which is additionally conducive to recovery.

Support During Recovery: Those who join the DNRS program gain access to a forum with others who are recovering from limbic system impairments. This is a very supportive environment, and one in which there is much support - both from coaches and other 'brain retrainers'. It is recommended to book a one to one Skype coaching session following completion of the DVD program so as to ensure a correct understanding of the program before beginning properly. This can be done via the DNRS website.

Oh, I'll just meditate - that will calm my limbic system down: Meditation may help to a degree, and in some cases may lead to recovery, but I do not think that, in general, it is powerful enough to *certainly* change limbic system function to the degree required. Furthermore, meditation does not change the limbic system in a targeted way. Rather, it creates 'psychological distance' between the person meditating and what is going on in the limbic system. Under normal circumstances, this can create calm but for someone with limbic system trauma it can make things worse as it is very difficult to gain 'psychological distance' from a brain in such distress. Indeed, meditation for those with limbic system trauma can actually increase distress as it is hard not to be 'sucked in' to the traumatic state the brain is in. The DNRS, on the other hand, is an intervention to change the limbic system itself, on its own terms and in deliberately positive directions, and is therefore more focussed on what is needed to rehabilitate the limbic system. After this rehabilitation has been completed, however, a more acceptance-based approach, as found in mindfulness, could be adopted.

Residual Anxieties / Release of Adrenalin After Recovery: Once the recovery process is complete, it is not uncommon - as with recovery from any health condition - to experience 'residual anxieties', i.e.: 'will my condition come back?' Fully recovered patients may feel 'remnants' of fear upon standing up, for example. Sometimes, these residual anxieties are amusing: a person may hear someone else talk about 'flower pots' and feel a twinge of anxiety (this frequently happens to the author of this book!). It is wise to see the humour in such anxieties and the best possible cure for them is consistently to engage in other activities, activities which take up your whole attention. Timetable your day to fill it with interesting activities of all sorts. Move away from non-anxious behaviour to normal behaviour and let the days pass. Do not preoccupy yourself with thoughts about health. Over time, your brain will forget these residual anxieties, as long as you keep it occupied for long enough with other things. I also note here that if the recovered person ever does start to feel adrenalin going off inappropriately and consistently, they should return for a few days to the DNRS exercises. A steady release of adrenalin over a few days will not damage the NET protein, but it is best - in the unlikely event this does happen - to cut it off in its tracks. As regards 'appropriate' adrenalin release in response to stressful situations, this should not be a cause for concern. Indeed, adrenalin is meant to help you cope with difficult situations! When it is not released as a result of an impairment, then adrenalin is your friend: use it to deal with the situation in front of you and get stuck in! Don't fall into the trap of thinking that adrenalin is in and of itself bad and don't fear its 'appropriate' release.

Cognitive Impairment: All POTS patients suffer from cognitive impairment - some to a considerable degree - and may find the DNRS exercises daunting as a result. The practice may feel 'murky' and 'cloudy' initially. This should not discourage the brain rewirer from continuing in her practice, however. Even a 'murky' DNRS practice is making the changes needed and, over time, this murkiness will recede as the limbic system starts to come out of a crisis state. Other changes such as giving up caffeine, sugar and perhaps limiting the use of technology, can all help with cognitive impairment.

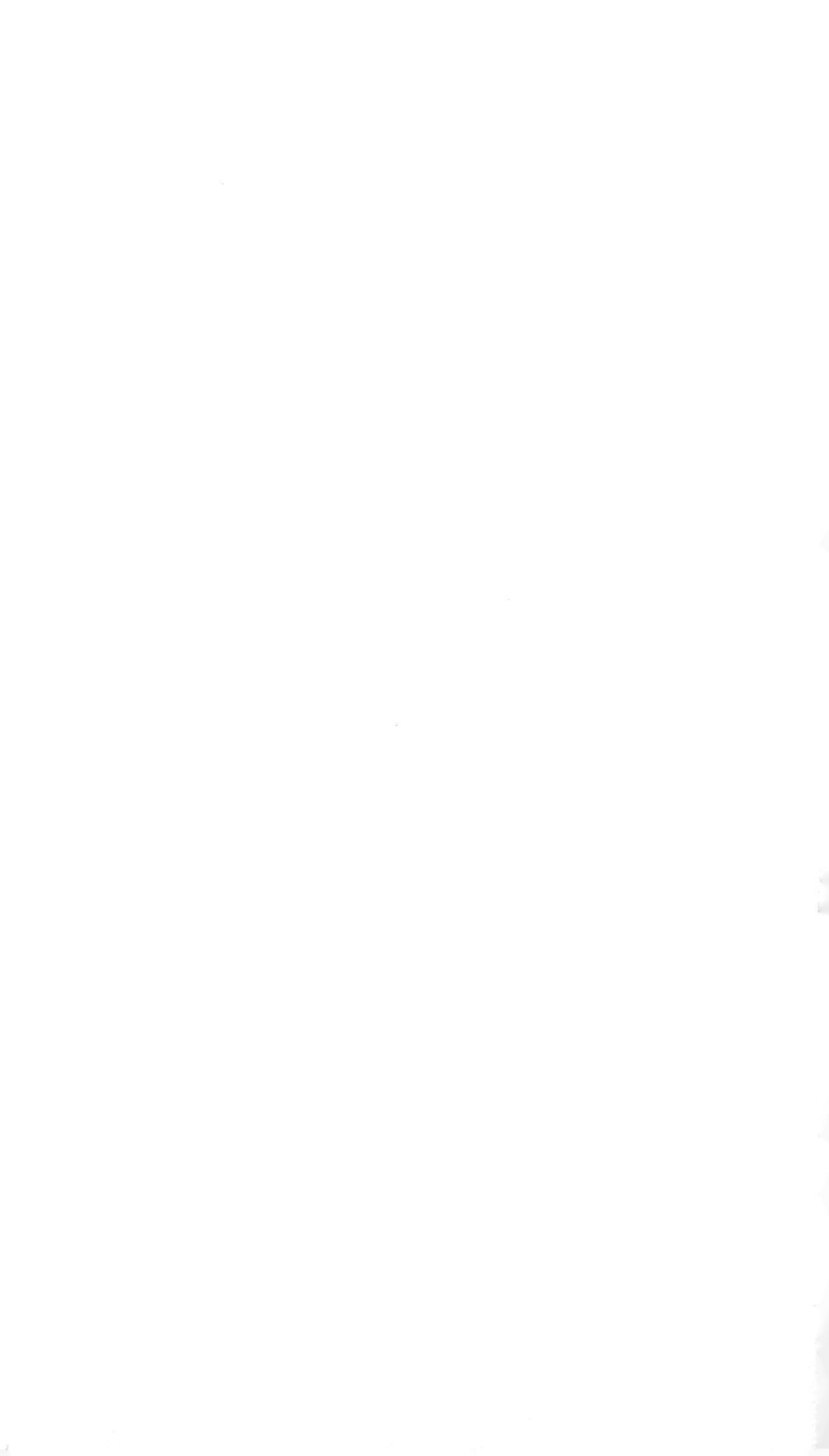

Printed in Great Britain
by Amazon